Independent BMTCN Study Guide:

850 Exam Style Practice Questions with Detailed Answer Explanations for the ONCC Blood and Marrow Transplant Certified Nurse Exam Prep

Caldwell Abiodun

Author Introduction

Certification as a **Blood and Marrow Transplant Certified Nurse (BMTCN®)** represents far more than professional advancement—it signifies a commitment to mastering one of the most complex and rapidly evolving specialties in nursing practice. The clinical demands of blood and marrow transplantation require not only technical precision but also a deep understanding of hematologic malignancies, cellular therapies, immunology, and the long-term management of vulnerable patient populations. This study guide was developed to support nurses preparing to meet that challenge with confidence and competence.

The author of this guide is an experienced transplant nursing professional who has dedicated years to caring for patients undergoing autologous and allogeneic blood and marrow transplantation across inpatient and outpatient settings. Working in collaboration with a team of transplant educators, advanced practice nurses, and certification-preparation specialists, the author brings together frontline clinical insight and evidence-based academic rigor. This combined expertise ensures that the content reflects both the realities of bedside practice and the expectations of the BMTCN® certification examination.

Throughout this guide, complex concepts—such as conditioning regimens, graft-versus-host disease, infection prevention, cellular therapy complications, and survivorship care—are presented with clarity and clinical relevance. The material is carefully aligned with the test blueprint, reinforcing critical thinking, patient safety principles, and the nuanced decision-making required in transplant environments. Special emphasis is placed on bridging theory to practice, enabling readers to apply knowledge directly to patient care scenarios they encounter daily.

Recognizing that nurses preparing for certification often balance demanding schedules and emotionally intensive work, this resource is structured for efficiency without sacrificing depth. High-yield summaries, practice-focused explanations, and integrated review strategies are designed to maximize retention while respecting the time constraints of working professionals. The goal is not only exam success, but strengthened clinical judgment and leadership within transplant teams.

Above all, this study guide reflects a steadfast belief in the transformative role of specialized nursing expertise. By pursuing BMTCN® certification, nurses affirm their dedication to excellence, advocacy, and lifelong learning. This guide stands as both a preparation tool and a professional companion—supporting candidates as they advance their knowledge, validate their skills, and continue delivering exceptional care to patients undergoing blood and marrow transplantation.

Table of Content

Disclaimer

Chapter 1: Foundations of Transplant

Blood and marrow transplantation rests on a deep understanding of cellular biology, immune function, and the therapeutic intent of hematopoietic reconstitution. Nurses in this specialty must integrate core scientific knowledge with patient-centered practice, translating complex biologic processes into effective clinical management and education.

According to the provided material, the field has advanced from its experimental roots in the mid-twentieth century to a mature therapy that relies on precise donor selection, conditioning regimens, and immune modulation. At the heart of the process is the hematopoietic stem cell, capable of regenerating all blood lineages after myeloablative or reduced-intensity therapy.

The goals of transplantation are multifaceted: to restore hematopoiesis, to replace diseased or defective marrow, and, in malignant disorders, to achieve a graft-versus-tumor effect. These cellular objectives guide treatment planning and post-transplant surveillance, shaping the nurse's role in both direct care and education.

Transplantation is also defined by its collaborative structure. Physicians, nurses, pharmacists, social workers, and dietitians contribute to a continuous cycle of preparation, infusion, and recovery. Within this team, the nurse maintains vigilance for physiologic instability while supporting psychosocial resilience, ensuring that the biologic foundations translate into safe and compassionate outcomes.

Hematopoietic Cell Lineage and Immune Function

All blood and immune cells derive from pluripotent hematopoietic stem cells housed primarily in the bone marrow. These progenitors differentiate into myeloid and lymphoid lineages, producing red blood cells, platelets, neutrophils, and lymphocytes that maintain oxygenation, coagulation, and defense.

In the transplant setting, the immune system is both a therapeutic ally and a potential source of complication. The graft-versus-tumor effect arises from donor lymphocytes recognizing malignant host cells as foreign, aiding in eradication of residual disease. Yet this same recognition underlies graft-versus-host disease (GVHD), a major source of morbidity.

For the nurse, understanding this duality is vital. Early indicators of immune reconstitution—such as neutrophil and platelet recovery—mark progress, but excessive immune activation or delayed recovery demands swift intervention. The interplay between engraftment, infection risk, and inflammatory response defines much of early post-transplant care.

Histocompatibility, particularly human leukocyte antigen (HLA) matching, determines the probability of graft acceptance. As explained in the clinical practice material, small molecular disparities between donor and recipient antigens can provoke rejection or severe GVHD. Modern matching techniques have greatly reduced these risks, but vigilance in education and monitoring remains essential.

Transplant Types, Indications, and Stem Cell Sources

Hematopoietic cell transplantation encompasses several modalities, each distinguished by the origin of stem cells and therapeutic intent.

Autologous transplantation involves harvesting the patient's own stem cells prior to high-dose therapy. It minimizes immune incompatibility but carries a risk of reinfusing malignant cells. **Allogeneic**

transplantation, by contrast, introduces donor cells, enabling both marrow restoration and immunologic tumor control through graft-versus-tumor mechanisms. Donor categories include matched related donors, matched unrelated donors, mismatched or haploidentical relatives, and umbilical cord blood units.

Emerging **cellular therapies**, such as CAR-T infusion, have expanded the transplant continuum by harnessing genetically modified immune cells to target specific malignancies. While distinct from traditional transplantation, these therapies require similar nursing competencies in cytokine monitoring, infection prevention, and patient education.

Stem cells may be obtained from peripheral blood, bone marrow, or umbilical cord sources. Each source influences engraftment kinetics and complication risk. Peripheral blood collection offers faster recovery but higher rates of chronic GVHD; marrow sources reduce GVHD but delay hematologic recovery. Nurses play a key role in patient and caregiver education regarding these trade-offs and in coordinating collection logistics with apheresis or surgical teams.

Recipient suitability depends on disease status, comorbidities, psychosocial readiness, and caregiver support. Comprehensive education for both patient and donor is central to ethical and successful outcomes, reinforcing informed consent and adherence throughout the transplant journey.

Recipient Suitability and Evaluation

Before a transplant is undertaken, a comprehensive evaluation determines the candidate's physical and psychosocial readiness. This process ensures that benefits outweigh risks and that recovery can be supported through both medical and personal resources.

Clinical assessment involves disease status, organ function, infection history, and prior therapy exposure. Laboratory evaluation typically includes hematologic panels, renal and hepatic profiles, and virologic screening. Imaging studies and pulmonary function tests establish baseline parameters for post-transplant comparison.

According to the reference materials, the evaluation extends beyond physiology. Transplant outcomes are heavily influenced by the individual's cognitive understanding, emotional resilience, and support network. The nurse contributes by assessing learning needs, coping strategies, and barriers to adherence. Collaborative discussions address fertility preservation, vaccination history, and psychosocial concerns such as caregiver availability or financial strain.

Through structured interviews and interdisciplinary rounds, the team ensures alignment between the patient's expectations and the procedure's realities. This foundation strengthens consent validity and reduces the likelihood of decisional regret. In practice, nurses often act as translators of complex medical information, converting clinical terminology into comprehensible, patient-centered dialogue.

Donor Selection, Care, and Education

Donor selection is guided primarily by histocompatibility, medical fitness, and willingness to participate. For allogeneic transplants, matching of HLA antigens across major loci—typically A, B, C, and DRB1—is critical. Even with improved technology, slight mismatches can provoke graft rejection or severe GVHD, making nurse-driven education on these processes essential to informed participation.

Donors, whether related or unrelated, undergo physical examinations, serologic testing, and counseling regarding the risks of collection procedures. Nurses coordinate scheduling, consent, and follow-up, ensuring that donors are medically cleared and emotionally supported. For peripheral blood collection, education focuses on mobilization agents, possible side effects, and post-apheresis care. Bone marrow donors are guided through anesthesia preparation and recovery expectations.

Ethical considerations—voluntary participation, confidentiality, and the right to withdraw—are emphasized throughout donor interactions. Education reinforces the altruistic nature of donation while acknowledging physical and psychological impacts. Nurses serve as advocates, balancing institutional needs with donor welfare, a principle reinforced in both European and North American transplant guidelines.

In cases involving umbilical cord blood, consent processes extend to the newborn's parents, requiring additional clarity on storage, ownership, and future use. Each donor encounter reflects the broader principle of respect for autonomy and commitment to transparent care.

Education and Interdisciplinary Preparation

Effective transplant care begins with education. Both recipients and caregivers must understand the trajectory of treatment—conditioning, infusion, isolation, engraftment, and recovery. Education plans should be iterative, revisited at every transition point, and customized to literacy level, culture, and emotional readiness.

Nursing education incorporates verbal explanation, written materials, and demonstration. Key topics include infection prevention, medication adherence, nutritional management, and early symptom reporting. Teaching also emphasizes self-care, fatigue management, and the importance of communication with the care team.

Interdisciplinary collaboration supports continuity: pharmacists review medication schedules, dietitians outline food safety and nutrition, and psychosocial specialists guide coping and support systems. The nurse acts as the anchor, ensuring that all teaching is synchronized and reinforced during inpatient and outpatient care.

Foundational preparation thus merges scientific precision with empathic practice. The nurse's ability to convey information clearly and compassionately reduces anxiety and enhances adherence. These educational foundations serve as the cornerstone upon which the entire transplant process—and the subsequent exam Chapters—are built.

Chapter 2: Transplant Process and Infusion

The transplant process integrates three major phases: **cell collection and storage**, **conditioning or preparative therapy**, and **cellular infusion**. Each requires strict adherence to timing, sterility, and multidisciplinary coordination.

From a nursing perspective, this Chapter translates complex protocols into consistent patient care. Understanding why each step occurs — and its potential complications — enables the nurse to anticipate clinical changes, reinforce safety procedures, and provide patient-centered explanations.

Stem cell collection begins once eligibility and donor compatibility are confirmed. Cells may be mobilized pharmacologically and collected via apheresis or harvested surgically from the marrow. The products are then processed, tested, and stored under cryogenic conditions until needed. Each specimen is uniquely identified and linked to recipient data to prevent mix-ups, following rigorous chain-of-custody verification.

Conditioning regimens immediately precede infusion and represent one of the most intensive aspects of care. They serve to eradicate malignant cells, suppress immunity, and create marrow space for engraftment. The nurse's role during this period is multifaceted: ensuring accurate administration, managing toxicity, monitoring organ function, and supporting comfort through symptom control and education.

Stem Cell Collection and Storage

Stem cell mobilization and collection demand exact coordination between medical, laboratory, and nursing teams. Mobilization agents, such as granulocyte colony-stimulating factors or chemotherapeutic adjuncts, stimulate progenitor cells to move from marrow to peripheral blood. The patient or donor is then connected to an apheresis machine that separates stem cells while returning other blood components.

Nurses monitor vital signs, calcium levels, and symptoms such as paresthesia or cramping related to citrate anticoagulation. Ongoing assessment ensures adequate collection volume and donor safety. Post-procedure care includes hydration, dietary reinforcement, and management of venipuncture sites or central line access.

Collected products are labeled and transported to processing laboratories where cell counts and sterility are verified. Cryopreservation techniques — commonly using dimethyl sulfoxide (DMSO) as a cryoprotectant — preserve cellular integrity. During freezing and thawing, strict temperature controls prevent damage. Nurses involved in this chain maintain awareness of contamination prevention, documentation accuracy, and regulatory compliance.

Storage may occur for weeks to months depending on clinical scheduling. The nurse's knowledge of handling procedures and emergency contingencies, such as equipment failure or accidental thawing, contributes directly to product viability and patient safety.

Conditioning and Infusion Management

Conditioning regimens combine chemotherapy, radiation, or targeted agents to prepare the recipient's marrow. The intensity may vary — myeloablative, reduced-intensity, or nonmyeloablative — depending on diagnosis, age, and comorbidities. Nurses monitor for acute toxicities including mucositis, nausea, hepatic dysfunction, and infection. Proactive symptom control preserves comfort and adherence.

Cellular infusion marks the transplant's pivotal moment. Cryopreserved stem cells are thawed at bedside or in controlled environments and infused intravenously, similar to a blood transfusion. Immediate nurse monitoring is critical: allergic reactions, hypertension, and DMSO-related effects such as bradycardia or garlic-like odor are possible. Oxygen saturation, blood pressure, and respiratory status must be observed continuously throughout and following the procedure.

The infusion nurse must also verify product identity, infusion rate, and line patency. Communication with the laboratory confirms product viability and infusion start times. Emotional support is equally significant; for many patients, this represents both a milestone and a moment of uncertainty. Providing calm explanations and reassurance sustains psychological safety during this transformative stage.

Following infusion, the focus shifts to engraftment monitoring and early complication management, establishing the bridge to the next Chapter.

Managing Complications of Conditioning Regimens

Conditioning therapy is a defining component of transplantation, and it is associated with significant toxicity risk. Chemotherapy, radiation, and biologic agents are administered in tightly controlled sequences to eliminate malignant cells and suppress host immunity. The nurse's role during this phase is continuous assessment, early recognition of complications, and prompt intervention.

Common acute effects include **mucositis**, **nausea and vomiting**, **diarrhea**, **fatigue**, **alopecia**, and **pancytopenia**. More severe reactions may involve **veno-occlusive disease (VOD)**, **pulmonary toxicity**, or **nephrotoxicity**. Monitoring includes daily weights, fluid balance, transaminases, and coagulation profiles to detect hepatic injury early.

Preventive care begins with hydration protocols, antiemetic regimens, and oral hygiene programs. Pain management for mucositis and infection prophylaxis for neutropenia are also key nursing interventions. Education reinforces dietary adjustments and adherence to mouth care routines to reduce bacterial load.

Radiation-based conditioning introduces unique safety considerations. Nurses must follow institutional protection policies and monitor for skin erythema, fatigue, and late-onset fibrosis. Close coordination with radiation therapy staff ensures accurate dose administration and minimal exposure outside the target field.

Infusion Management and Adverse Reactions

The infusion phase requires uninterrupted vigilance. Prior to starting, the nurse performs **double verification** of patient identity, product label, and ABO compatibility. A pre-infusion assessment establishes baseline temperature, blood pressure, pulse, respiratory rate, and oxygen saturation.

During infusion, side effects may appear abruptly. **DMSO toxicity** from cryopreserved products can cause chest tightness, nausea, or hypotension; patients often report a garlic or oyster odor on the breath. Nurses manage these effects with rate adjustment, supplemental oxygen, or antihistamines as ordered.

Allergic or anaphylactoid reactions may occur in response to cellular or plasma proteins. The nurse keeps emergency equipment at bedside and maintains direct visual contact with the patient for the first fifteen minutes. **Bradycardia, dyspnea, or urticaria** warrant immediate pause and notification of the transplant physician.

Post-infusion observation continues for several hours. Documentation must include start and completion times, total volume infused, product identification numbers, and any adverse events. Patient reassurance and explanation of expected sensations promote calm and cooperation. Emotional support remains a vital nursing contribution during what many recipients view as their "new marrow birthday."

Cellular Therapies Beyond Standard Infusion

Modern hematology has expanded transplantation into the field of **cellular therapy**, where modified immune cells are administered for targeted disease control. Among these, **donor lymphocyte infusions (DLI)** and **chimeric antigen receptor T-cell (CAR-T)** therapies are most clinically established.

DLI is used post-allogeneic transplant to enhance graft-versus-tumor activity or reverse relapse. Nursing care emphasizes close monitoring for cytopenias, infection, and **GVHD** development, which can occur days to weeks later. Education focuses on symptom recognition—particularly skin rash, diarrhea, or jaundice—as early indicators requiring urgent evaluation.

CAR-T therapy employs autologous T-cells engineered to recognize tumor-specific antigens. Nurses must be proficient in detecting **cytokine release syndrome (CRS)** and **immune effector cell-associated neurotoxicity syndrome (ICANS)**. Early manifestations include fever, hypotension, or confusion. Prompt escalation of care, fluid support, and adherence to institutional response algorithms are lifesaving measures.

These therapies bridge traditional transplantation and immunotherapy, reinforcing the need for BMTCN-certified nurses to remain at the forefront of rapidly evolving practice. Safety, education, and interdisciplinary communication remain central to all cellular therapy care.

Chapter 3: Early Post-Transplant Management and Education

The early post-transplant phase begins immediately following cellular infusion and extends through initial engraftment and immune recovery. During this time, patients are profoundly immunocompromised, often cytopenic, and at risk for a broad spectrum of complications.

Nursing priorities include **infection prevention**, **immune suppression management**, **hematologic recovery monitoring**, and **education for symptom awareness**. Vigilant assessment—hourly in the acute phase—is essential. Subtle changes in temperature, blood pressure, or mental status may signal infection or inflammatory response.

According to the provided materials, interdisciplinary coordination is essential in this period. Pharmacists guide antimicrobial prophylaxis; dietitians ensure neutropenic diet compliance; physical therapists prevent deconditioning. The nurse acts as the hub for this collaboration, maintaining consistent communication among disciplines and providing continuous patient updates.

Family education is equally crucial. Caregivers must understand isolation precautions, hand hygiene, and visitation limits. The nurse's communication reinforces that these measures are protective rather than restrictive, helping reduce the psychological burden of isolation for both patient and family.

Immunosuppressive Therapy and Acute GVHD

Immunosuppressive therapy prevents graft rejection and moderates donor immune cell activity. Common agents include calcineurin inhibitors, antimetabolites, and corticosteroids. The nurse monitors drug levels, renal and hepatic function, and early signs of toxicity such as hypertension, tremor, or mucosal ulceration.

Adherence education forms a cornerstone of this Chapter. Patients must understand that missed or mistimed doses may precipitate graft rejection or severe graft-versus-host disease (GVHD). Teaching includes timing consistency, drug–food interactions, and symptom reporting for potential side effects.

Acute GVHD typically manifests within the first 100 days post-transplant, affecting skin, liver, and gastrointestinal tract. Early signs include rash, bilirubin elevation, and diarrhea. Nursing assessment relies on meticulous documentation of skin integrity, stool volume, and hepatic function tests. Prompt reporting leads to timely therapeutic adjustment, often involving corticosteroids or targeted immunosuppressive infusions.

Education continues even during flare management. Patients and caregivers must recognize that GVHD control balances suppression of donor activity with preservation of anti-tumor benefit. Emotional reassurance is vital—many patients fear GVHD as failure, while in fact controlled immune activation can correlate with improved relapse outcomes.

Infection Prevention, Sepsis, and Early Complications

Profound neutropenia and mucosal disruption render patients vulnerable to bacterial, viral, and fungal pathogens. Nursing vigilance includes **aseptic technique**, **environmental control**, and **prompt fever management**. Central line maintenance, daily line assessment, and chlorhexidine site care reduce bloodstream infection risk.

When fever occurs, nurses initiate sepsis protocols without delay—obtaining cultures, administering empiric antibiotics, and monitoring hemodynamics. Timely action within the first hour of recognition markedly improves survival. Education for caregivers includes recognizing fever thresholds (≥100.4°F / 38°C) and the importance of avoiding over-the-counter antipyretics before reporting symptoms.

Other early complications include **pancytopenia**, **transfusion support needs**, and **nutritional deficits**. Nurses coordinate blood component therapy, observe for transfusion reactions, and ensure prophylactic platelet thresholds are maintained. Nutritional collaboration maintains protein intake and electrolyte balance critical for tissue repair.

Psychological strain is also intense during this phase. Anxiety, sleep disruption, and adjustment reactions are common. Incorporating psychosocial check-ins within routine assessments ensures comprehensive care and supports emotional stability during the most vulnerable post-infusion period.

Immune Reconstitution and Hematologic Recovery

Following transplantation, immune recovery unfolds gradually as donor-derived hematopoietic stem cells repopulate marrow and restore functional immunity. Nurses monitor laboratory markers of engraftment such as **absolute neutrophil count (ANC)**, **platelet recovery**, and **chimerism levels**.

Engraftment typically occurs within two to four weeks for peripheral blood sources and slightly later for marrow or cord blood. During this time, the patient remains at risk for infection and inflammatory syndromes such as **engraftment syndrome** and **cytokine release syndrome (CRS)**.

Engraftment syndrome manifests as fever, rash, and weight gain linked to capillary leak. Nurses respond with careful fluid monitoring, administration of corticosteroids as prescribed, and supportive oxygen or diuretics. CRS, often associated with immune effector cell therapies, presents similarly but can escalate to hypotension and hypoxia. Early detection and adherence to escalation algorithms are lifesaving.

Immune reconstitution continues for months, guided by prophylactic antimicrobial therapy and revaccination schedules. Nurses play a vital educational role, reinforcing medication adherence, infection avoidance, and environmental precautions such as avoiding live plants, standing water, and crowded spaces during early recovery.

Nutritional Support and System-Specific Complications

Nutrition profoundly influences recovery. The combination of mucositis, nausea, altered taste, and anorexia often leads to caloric deficit and delayed healing. Nurses collaborate with dietitians to develop individualized meal plans emphasizing high-protein, small, frequent meals and adequate hydration.

When oral intake is inadequate, **enteral feeding** is preferred to preserve gut integrity; **parenteral nutrition** is reserved for severe gastrointestinal dysfunction. Continuous monitoring of electrolytes, glucose tolerance, and liver enzymes ensures safety during supplementation. Education includes maintaining food safety—avoiding raw foods, unpasteurized products, and cross-contamination—to reduce infection risk.

System-specific complications demand focused nursing assessment.

- **Hepatic veno-occlusive disease (VOD):** monitored via weight gain, hepatomegaly, and jaundice; prevention relies on judicious fluid balance and early symptom recognition.

- **Pulmonary toxicity:** nurses assess breath sounds and oxygenation, noting any dyspnea or cough as potential early signs.
- **Renal dysfunction:** may result from calcineurin inhibitors or sepsis; careful I&O and medication adjustment collaboration are essential.

These physiologic complications are often interrelated, requiring nurses to integrate data from multiple systems and anticipate cascading effects such as fluid overload or multi-organ stress.

Symptom Management and Patient Education

Symptom management is the unifying thread of early post-transplant nursing. Pain, nausea, fatigue, and anxiety occur in overlapping cycles. Nurses employ pharmacologic and nonpharmacologic strategies—antiemetics, relaxation techniques, music therapy, and energy conservation—to enhance comfort and adherence.

Fatigue remains one of the most reported symptoms. Encouraging paced activity, adequate rest, and gradual mobilization preserves functional status. Regular evaluation using standardized scales helps guide individualized interventions.

Education at this phase centers on recognizing concerning signs—persistent fever, uncontrolled pain, bleeding, or confusion—and understanding when to seek immediate help. Reinforcing medication schedules, infection precautions, and hydration targets empowers patients and caregivers to participate actively in recovery.

In all aspects of symptom management, nurses balance vigilance with empathy. By normalizing the emotional strain and validating patient experiences, they transform technical expertise into human-centered healing. This integrated model of symptom care lays the groundwork for the transition to late post-transplant management.

Download Audio file and flashcards

Chapter 4: Late Post-Transplant Management and Education

The late post-transplant period begins approximately 100 days after infusion, extending into long-term survivorship. During this phase, the patient transitions from acute monitoring to sustained health maintenance, requiring coordinated follow-up between the transplant center, primary care, and subspecialists.

Major priorities include **management of chronic GVHD**, **monitoring for late effects**, **infection prevention**, and **disease surveillance**. Nurses continue to act as educators and advocates, guiding patients through changing therapy regimens and lifestyle adjustments.

Chronic GVHD affects multiple organ systems and can persist for months or years. Late effects of therapy—such as cataracts, infertility, endocrine dysfunction, and secondary malignancies—reflect the lasting cellular impact of conditioning regimens and immune suppression. Ongoing assessment ensures early identification and mitigation.

Long-term recovery also introduces new psychosocial challenges. As patients re-enter work or social settings, fatigue, anxiety, and fear of relapse can resurface. Nursing care balances physical assessment with emotional support, fostering resilience and a sense of restored normalcy.

Chronic GVHD and System-Specific Late Effects

Chronic GVHD remains one of the most complex post-transplant conditions, involving the skin, liver, lungs, and mucous membranes. It can mimic autoimmune disorders, presenting with dryness, rash, fibrosis, or joint restriction. Nurses assess symptom patterns, document severity, and ensure adherence to immunosuppressive therapy and topical treatments.

Management requires coordination across specialties—dermatology for skin involvement, ophthalmology for ocular dryness, and pulmonology for bronchiolitis obliterans. **Photopheresis** and targeted biologic therapies have improved outcomes, but nursing follow-up ensures safety and continuity. Education emphasizes sun protection, skin hydration, and infection vigilance.

System-specific late effects extend beyond GVHD. Radiation and chemotherapy may cause endocrine disruption, infertility, and metabolic syndromes. Nurses monitor hormonal levels, counsel on fertility preservation options prior to transplant, and refer to reproductive specialists when appropriate. Cardiac and pulmonary screening is ongoing, as late-onset fibrosis or cardiomyopathy can appear years after treatment.

Through compassionate engagement and clinical precision, the nurse helps patients navigate the balance between surveillance and normal life, ensuring adherence without fostering excessive fear.

Infection Prevention, Relapse, and Follow-Up Care

Even after immune recovery, transplant recipients remain vulnerable to infection due to incomplete vaccine response and ongoing immunosuppressive therapy. Revaccination protocols usually begin six months post-transplant and include inactivated vaccines first, followed by live vaccines after immune competency is confirmed. Nurses ensure adherence to vaccination schedules and reinforce daily hygiene and food safety practices.

Relapse monitoring is central to long-term follow-up. Patients with malignant disorders undergo routine blood counts, bone marrow assessments, and molecular testing. Nurses interpret trends, track symptoms such as unexplained fatigue or lymphadenopathy, and facilitate rapid re-evaluation if relapse indicators appear.

Follow-up care incorporates milestone visits at defined intervals—commonly 3, 6, 12 months, and annually thereafter. These visits include organ-specific screening, psychosocial evaluation, and survivorship planning. The nurse plays a pivotal role in coordinating appointments, reviewing medications, and reinforcing health maintenance behaviors such as exercise, smoking cessation, and balanced nutrition.

Secondary Malignancies and Disease Relapse

Late complications of transplantation may include **secondary malignancies**, arising from prior chemotherapy, radiation exposure, or prolonged immunosuppression. These conditions represent a small but serious risk that requires lifelong vigilance. Nurses educate survivors on self-examination, symptom awareness, and the importance of routine cancer screenings such as mammography, dermatologic evaluations, and colonoscopy.

Hematologic relapses—such as leukemia recurrence—demand prompt recognition. Early indicators may appear as cytopenias, abnormal peripheral smears, or subtle changes in well-being. Nurses reviewing laboratory results must correlate findings with the patient's baseline trajectory and escalate deviations promptly.

When relapse occurs, management options include donor lymphocyte infusion, targeted therapies, or a second transplant. The emotional impact can be profound; the nurse's role extends beyond physical support to providing compassionate communication, reinforcing hope without minimizing reality. Education emphasizes that relapse management is an active, multi-step process, not an endpoint.

Surveillance also involves regular assessment for precancerous conditions such as oral leukoplakia or human papillomavirus (HPV)-related changes. A preventive mindset, grounded in teaching and empowerment, sustains the patient's engagement with long-term wellness.

Long-Term Surveillance and Health Maintenance

Long-term follow-up clinics provide structure for ongoing assessment. Visits typically include laboratory evaluation, pulmonary and cardiac screening, endocrine function testing, and vaccination review. The nurse's responsibilities include ensuring continuity of care between the transplant center and community providers, maintaining updated medication lists, and confirming adherence to recommended monitoring schedules.

Common late health maintenance focuses include:

- **Endocrine and metabolic health:** screening for hypothyroidism, diabetes, dyslipidemia, and bone loss; advocating for adequate calcium and vitamin D intake.
- **Cardiopulmonary function:** monitoring for late-onset cardiomyopathy or restrictive lung disease through echocardiography and pulmonary testing.

- **Neurocognitive function:** observing for memory or concentration issues, often related to prior chemotherapy or total body irradiation.

Health promotion becomes central in this phase. Nurses encourage survivors to engage in physical activity suited to their tolerance, practice infection prevention, and adhere to balanced nutrition. Counseling around alcohol, smoking, and sun exposure prevention reinforces overall well-being.

A hallmark of expert nursing practice is recognizing subtle patterns—declining stamina, recurrent infections, or mood changes—that may signal emerging chronic complications. Continuous advocacy ensures that no aspect of survivorship is overlooked.

Survivorship and Transition of Care

Survivorship marks the shift from acute medical dependence to sustained self-management. It involves physical, psychological, social, and spiritual dimensions. According to the provided reference material, structured survivorship programs improve adherence, reduce distress, and empower patients to reclaim daily routines.

Nurses facilitate this transition by developing individualized **survivorship care plans** summarizing treatment history, potential late effects, and recommended follow-up. These plans bridge communication between oncology teams, primary care, and the patient, ensuring continuity and informed participation in health decisions.

Psychosocial adaptation varies; some survivors experience gratitude and renewed purpose, while others struggle with fatigue, anxiety, or post-traumatic stress symptoms. The nurse integrates supportive counseling, referral to survivorship groups, and mindfulness or coping strategies tailored to patient preference.

Spiritual well-being is often revisited during recovery. Encouraging reflection, legacy-building, and reconnection with life goals reinforces meaning beyond survival. The holistic approach—addressing both body and spirit—embodies the professional standard expected of BMTCN-certified nurses.

Chapter 5: Quality of Life

Psychosocial and Emotional Support

Quality of life in transplant nursing extends beyond survival. It includes emotional adaptation, family cohesion, and restoration of daily identity. The psychological toll of transplantation is considerable—patients experience prolonged isolation, loss of independence, and fear of relapse. Nurses address these needs through empathetic communication, structured emotional assessment, and linkage to supportive counseling.

Psychosocial interventions begin early and continue across recovery. Encouraging expression of fears, normalizing mood fluctuations, and facilitating peer or survivor group contact build resilience. According to the provided material, open dialogue between patient, family, and care team improves adherence and satisfaction. Nurses also watch for depression, anxiety, or cognitive changes that may indicate adjustment disorder or medication side effects.

Family caregivers often endure comparable stress. Teaching coping techniques, scheduling rest, and validating their role sustain the support network that underpins recovery. In this way, psychosocial care is inseparable from clinical excellence—it is the human counterpart to scientific precision.

Cultural, Spiritual, and Health Promotion Dimensions

Cultural competence ensures that care respects beliefs, language, and values influencing decision-making and health behavior. Transplant nurses engage interpreters when needed, avoid assumptions about family roles, and adapt education materials for literacy and cultural context. Understanding dietary customs, spiritual rituals, and alternative health practices fosters trust and adherence.

Spiritual care complements psychological well-being. Many patients seek meaning in their illness or recovery; others draw strength from prayer, meditation, or community faith leaders. Nurses facilitate access to chaplaincy and encourage self-defined spiritual expression. Presence and active listening often provide the greatest comfort, affirming dignity throughout recovery.

Health promotion extends into lifestyle restoration—encouraging graded exercise, balanced diet, and stress-reduction practices. Smoking cessation, alcohol moderation, and safe sun exposure are standard counseling points. Teaching self-monitoring for fatigue, infection signs, and emotional distress reinforces patient empowerment, transforming recovery into active wellness rather than passive survival.

Palliative and End-of-Life Care

Despite medical progress, some transplant recipients experience irreversible complications or relapse. Integrating **palliative care** early enhances comfort and dignity while supporting decision-making. Nurses identify symptom burden—pain, dyspnea, nausea, and anxiety—and collaborate with interdisciplinary teams for optimal control.

Palliative engagement does not signal failure; it redefines success as relief of suffering and alignment with patient values. When prognosis becomes limited, nurses guide families through discussions on **advance directives**, hospice resources, and legacy-building. Maintaining transparency and compassion fosters trust and allows for peaceful closure.

Even in terminal phases, nurses sustain the therapeutic relationship by honoring patient autonomy and cultural preferences. Moments of presence—holding a hand, listening without judgment, respecting silence—become as vital as any pharmacologic intervention.

By uniting curative and palliative philosophies, the BMTCN-certified nurse ensures continuity of dignity across the entire transplant continuum.

Chapter 6: Professional Performance

Professional practice in blood and marrow transplantation is grounded in established standards that ensure consistency, quality, and accountability. The **Oncology Nursing Certification Corporation (ONCC)** framework emphasizes safe, evidence-based, and ethically sound care. Within this framework, BMTCN®-certified nurses apply clinical judgment to every step of the transplant process—from pre-transplant assessment through survivorship.

Standards of care include accurate assessment, timely intervention, documentation integrity, and advocacy for patient rights. Nurses are expected to maintain competence through continuing education, participation in quality improvement initiatives, and engagement in professional organizations such as transplant or oncology nursing networks.

Standards of professional performance extend beyond bedside care. They encompass contributions to evidence-based practice, mentorship of peers, participation in policy development, and commitment to lifelong learning. The professional nurse exemplifies reliability, compassion, and interdisciplinary respect, modeling ethical and clinical excellence for the healthcare team.

Adherence to standards fosters not only regulatory compliance but also trust—a cornerstone of the therapeutic relationship and an expectation of certification-level practice.

Leadership, Collaboration, and Quality Improvement

Effective transplant nursing depends on collaboration among physicians, pharmacists, social workers, and laboratory staff. The nurse often coordinates the flow of information and interventions, ensuring patient needs remain central amid complex protocols.

Leadership in this environment is not confined to administrative roles; it manifests through advocacy, teaching, and consistent role modeling. A nurse who identifies a safety gap and initiates a corrective process demonstrates professional leadership in action.

Quality improvement (QI) and **evidence-based practice (EBP)** are essential extensions of leadership. QI projects might evaluate infection rates, line maintenance compliance, or patient education outcomes. Incorporating EBP ensures that every intervention reflects current research and clinical consensus.

Interdisciplinary collaboration promotes comprehensive care. Regular communication rounds, shared decision-making, and transparent documentation prevent duplication and error. By fostering collegial respect, nurses contribute to team cohesion—a predictor of better patient outcomes.

In high-acuity transplant units, leadership also involves crisis management. The nurse's calm presence during emergencies guides team response and reassures patients and families, underscoring the influence of professional demeanor on therapeutic success.

Ethics, Legal Considerations, and Accreditation

Transplantation presents unique ethical and legal challenges. Nurses uphold **autonomy, beneficence, nonmaleficence, and justice**, ensuring that care aligns with patient values and informed consent. Ethical dilemmas may include donor risk versus recipient benefit, experimental therapy participation, or allocation of scarce resources.

Legal responsibilities include accurate documentation, adherence to privacy laws, and maintaining clear professional boundaries. Nurses must recognize potential conflicts of interest and ensure confidentiality in all donor and recipient interactions. Informed consent is a continuous process—not a single signature—and nurses reinforce understanding at each stage of care.

Accreditation and regulatory standards, such as those set by the **Foundation for the Accreditation of Cellular Therapy (FACT)** and **The Joint Commission**, define operational excellence in transplant programs. Nurses support compliance by maintaining documentation accuracy, adhering to safety protocols, and participating in institutional audits.

Self-care also constitutes an ethical responsibility. Compassion fatigue and burnout are genuine risks in this demanding specialty. Regular reflection, peer support, and utilization of employee wellness programs preserve the resilience necessary for sustained professional excellence.

Evidence-Based Practice and Research Integration

Advancing transplant nursing requires the ongoing application of research and the integration of emerging evidence into clinical protocols. **Evidence-based practice (EBP)** ensures that interventions reflect the most current understanding of effectiveness and safety. Nurses critically appraise literature, participate in data collection, and translate findings into daily care strategies.

Research in transplantation frequently explores infection control, symptom management, psychosocial outcomes, and cellular therapy innovations. Nurses contribute by identifying clinical questions, supporting study enrollment, and maintaining ethical standards in human subject protection. Accurate data recording and informed consent processes safeguard both participants and institutional integrity.

Participation in professional conferences, journal clubs, and collaborative projects fosters a culture of curiosity and learning. The professional nurse not only applies evidence but also helps generate it—bridging the gap between bedside observation and published advancement. This engagement enhances personal competence and elevates the field as a whole.

Communication, Collaboration, and Interdisciplinary Practice

Clear, respectful communication forms the foundation of safe and effective transplant care. Transplant patients interact with large, multidisciplinary teams—oncologists, infectious disease specialists, pharmacists, dietitians, and psychosocial staff. The nurse ensures coordination among these professionals through concise handoffs, timely updates, and unified care plans.

SBAR (Situation, Background, Assessment, Recommendation) frameworks are widely adopted to standardize communication and minimize error. Regular interdisciplinary rounds and patient-care conferences further reinforce alignment across the team.

Nurses also cultivate therapeutic communication with patients and families. Active listening, empathy, and honesty build trust—particularly when discussing complex topics such as prognosis, side effects, or ethical dilemmas. By acknowledging patient emotions and providing clarity, the nurse becomes both advocate and guide.

Cultural sensitivity remains integral to collaboration. Awareness of differing decision-making styles, family hierarchies, and communication norms ensures inclusivity. As bridge-builders, nurses translate medical language into understandable information, empowering patients to participate meaningfully in their care.

Environmental Safety, Resource Utilization, and Self-Care

The transplant environment requires strict adherence to infection control and safety standards. Personal protective equipment (PPE), isolation protocols, and aseptic technique protect both patient and healthcare team. Nurses verify equipment integrity, ensure negative-pressure room functionality, and participate in periodic safety audits.

Resource utilization involves balancing quality with efficiency. Nurses coordinate scheduling, reduce redundant testing, and manage supply usage responsibly while maintaining patient-centered priorities. Awareness of institutional budgets does not diminish advocacy; rather, it refines decision-making to achieve sustainable excellence.

Equally vital is **self-care**. The emotional demands of transplant nursing can lead to compassion fatigue and burnout. Strategies such as mindfulness, debriefing sessions, adequate rest, and professional boundary maintenance preserve resilience. Institutions increasingly recognize self-care as a quality measure—healthy nurses deliver safer, more empathetic care.

By safeguarding both environment and self, the nurse sustains the integrity of the profession. The capacity to care for others begins with caring for oneself, embodying the ethical principle of respect for all human well-being—including the caregiver's own.

Chapter 7 – Practice Question and Answers

Questions (1-100)

Q1. A 62-year-old patient with relapsed multiple myeloma is being evaluated for autologous hematopoietic stem cell transplant. Which stem cell source is most commonly used for autologous transplants?

A. Bone marrow
B. Peripheral blood stem cells
C. Umbilical cord blood
D. Placental stem cells

Q2. Which HLA locus is primarily involved in antigen presentation to CD8+ T cells?

A. HLA-DR
B. HLA-DQ
C. HLA-A
D. HLA-DP

Q3. A patient is scheduled for allogeneic transplant from a sibling. Which donor type best describes a fully HLA-matched sibling?

A. Matched unrelated donor (MURD)
B. Matched related donor (MRD)
C. Haploidentical donor
D. Mismatched unrelated donor

Q4. Which cellular goal of allogeneic transplant most directly contributes to long-term control of hematologic malignancy?

A. Rapid neutrophil recovery
B. Graft-versus-tumor (GvT) effect
C. Avoidance of transfusion dependence
D. Prevention of mucositis

Q5. Which lab test is most directly used to quantify CD34+ progenitor cells before collection?

A. Flow cytometry on peripheral blood
B. CBC with differential
C. Serum ferritin
D. Peripheral blood culture

Q6. Which indication is a well-established hematologic reason for hematopoietic cell transplantation?

A. Early-stage localized prostate cancer
B. Severe aplastic anemia refractory to immunosuppression
C. Uncomplicated iron deficiency anemia
D. Stable chronic osteoarthritis

Q7. In the context of donor selection for unrelated donors, which organization maintains large volunteer donor registries internationally?

A. CIBMTR
B. WMDA
C. ASBMT
D. NCI

Q8. Which preparative regimen term best describes an approach designed to suppress immunity enough to allow donor engraftment without fully ablating host marrow?

A. Myeloablative
B. Total marrow ablation
C. Hematopoietic rescue

D. Non-myeloablative

Q9. Which cell lineage originates from a common myeloid progenitor?

A. T lymphocytes
B. Erythrocytes
C. B lymphocytes
D. Natural killer cells

Q10. Which graft type most commonly carries higher risk of chronic GVHD in adults?

A. Umbilical cord blood
B. Peripheral blood stem cell grafts
C. Autologous grafts
D. Cryopreserved platelet transfusion

Q11. A 45-year-old candidate has uncontrolled severe heart failure. Regarding recipient suitability, which statement is most appropriate?

A. Uncontrolled severe heart failure is a contraindication to transplant until optimized.
B. Cardiac status is not considered in transplant eligibility.
C. Active heart failure improves transplant outcomes.
D. Heart failure is only relevant post-transplant.

Q12. Which feature of umbilical cord blood grafts explains their relative tolerance of greater HLA mismatch?

A. Higher CD34+ count than PBSC
B. Naïve immune cell phenotype with reduced alloreactivity
C. Robust adult memory T-cell content
D. Permanent adult donor chimerism

Q13. Which educational priority is most important for a recipient prior to discharge after transplant conditioning?

A. Detailed genomic testing methods
B. Infection prevention and when to contact the transplant team
C. Advanced radiotherapy techniques
D. Laboratory instrument calibration

Q14. Which component of the immune system is primarily responsible for immediate defense against encapsulated bacteria after transplant?

A. CD8+ T lymphocytes
B. Complement and neutrophils
C. Bone remnant stromal cells
D. Erythrocytes

Q15. Which donor factor most increases the risk of graft-versus-host disease in allogeneic transplant recipients?

A. Donor ABO mismatch
B. Donor parity status irrelevant
C. Higher donor T-cell dose in the graft
D. Donor age less than recipient age always reduces GVHD

Q16. Which component of pre-transplant evaluation assesses infectious risk related to latent viruses?

A. Pulmonary function tests
B. Serologic testing for CMV, EBV, and hepatitis
C. Echocardiogram for ejection fraction
D. Bone density scan

Q17. Which statement best describes chimerism monitoring after allogeneic transplant?

A. It quantifies proportions of donor versus recipient hematopoiesis to assess engraftment.

B. It measures only cytokine levels.
C. It is unnecessary clinically.
D. It is used solely to assess renal function.

Q18. Which preparative agent class is most associated with mucosal barrier injury (mucositis) when used at high doses?

A. Alkylating agents (e.g., busulfan, cyclophosphamide)
B. Oral antihistamines
C. Topical emollients
D. Intranasal vaccines

Q19. Who should receive education about caregiving and infection precautions before donor stem cell collection and transplant?

A. Only the patient
B. Patient and primary caregiver(s)
C. Spectators in the waiting room
D. Transplant team only

Q20. Which biologic therapy is considered a cellular therapy distinct from traditional HSCT and may be listed separately on the BMTCN outline?

A. CAR-T cell therapy
B. Oral azithromycin prophylaxis
C. Topical steroid cream
D. Routine influenza vaccination

Q21. Which organ produces erythropoietin, the hormone responsible for red cell production?

A. Liver
B. Kidney
C. Spleen
D. Bone marrow

Q22. Which major immune cell population is central to graft-versus-host disease?

A. $CD8^{+}$ cytotoxic T cells
B. Neutrophils
C. Platelets
D. Erythrocytes

Q23. Which disease is least likely to be treated with hematopoietic stem cell transplantation?

A. Acute myeloid leukemia
B. Multiple myeloma
C. Chronic obstructive pulmonary disease
D. Severe aplastic anemia

Q24. Which best describes "haploidentical" donor–recipient matching?

A. Identical at all HLA loci
B. Completely mismatched
C. Matched at half of HLA alleles (one haplotype)
D. Matched only for ABO group

Q25. The primary function of $CD4^{+}$ T helper cells post-transplant is to:

A. Produce erythropoietin
B. Enhance B-cell antibody production and immune coordination
C. Phagocytose pathogens
D. Form platelet aggregates

Q26. Which factor most directly influences donor selection for related donors?

A. ABO typing alone

B. HLA matching results
C. Serum creatinine level of recipient
D. Donor age difference > 10 years

Q27. Which hematopoietic stem cell surface marker is used to identify transplantable cells?
A. CD4
B. CD8
C. CD34
D. CD19

Q28. Why is peripheral blood favored over marrow as a stem cell source for autologous transplants?
A. Simpler cryopreservation
B. Faster engraftment and shorter neutropenia
C. Lower $CD34^+$ count
D. Reduced mobilization costs

Q29. Which immunologic concept explains how allogeneic grafts can control malignancy after transplant?
A. Central tolerance
B. Clonal anergy
C. Graft-versus-tumor (GvT) effect
D. Peripheral tolerance

Q30. During stem cell mobilization, G-CSF acts by:
A. Inhibiting stem cell release from marrow
B. Stimulating progenitor release into peripheral blood
C. Inducing apoptosis of stem cells
D. Blocking bone marrow stromal adhesion molecules

Q31. A donor education session should include discussion of:
A. Potential apheresis side effects and post-donation care
B. Recipient's diagnosis in detail
C. Hospital billing systems
D. Nutrition guidelines for recipients

Q32. Which HLA class II molecule is most important for $CD4^+$ T-cell antigen presentation?
A. HLA-A
B. HLA-B
C. HLA-DR
D. HLA-C

Q33. Which stem cell source requires cryopreservation most often before infusion?
A. Fresh bone marrow
B. Peripheral blood autograft
C. Umbilical cord blood
D. Haploidentical bone marrow

Q34. In which scenario is an autologous transplant contraindicated?
A. Acute myeloid leukemia with marrow involvement
B. Lymphoma in remission
C. Multiple myeloma first response
D. Relapsed testicular cancer

Q35. Which term describes replacement of host hematopoiesis by donor cells after transplant?
A. Engraftment
B. Apoptosis
C. Degranulation

D. Fibrinolysis

Q36. Which pre-transplant test assesses lung tolerance to conditioning regimens?

A. EEG
B. Abdominal ultrasound
C. Bone scan
D. Pulmonary function tests (PFTs)

Q37. Which parameter defines successful neutrophil engraftment after allogeneic HSCT?

A. ANC > 500/µL for 3 consecutive days
B. Platelet count > 100,000/µL
C. WBC < 1,000/µL
D. $CD34^+$ count > 2×10^6/kg collected

Q38. During patient education on stem cell collection, which topic is most critical?

A. Need for adequate hydration and calcium monitoring during apheresis
B. The recipient's HLA typing algorithm
C. Hospital billing codes
D. Cryopreservation machine settings

Q39. In hematopoiesis, which cell type is the direct precursor to platelets?

A. Myeloblast
B. Megakaryocyte
C. Monocyte
D. Eosinophil

Q40. Which statement best characterizes CAR-T cell therapy relative to HSCT?

A. It uses genetically modified autologous T cells targeting specific antigens.
B. It is a form of high-dose chemotherapy without cells.
C. It requires donor stem cell infusion for engraftment.
D. It cannot treat hematologic malignancies.

Q41. Which of the following is the primary method for assessing donor-recipient HLA compatibility in allogeneic hematopoietic stem cell transplantation?

A. Serum glucose levels
B. HLA typing
C. Peripheral blood culture
D. Bone marrow biopsy

Q42. Which cell lineage is responsible for producing platelets in the bone marrow?

A. Erythroid precursors
B. Myeloid precursors
C. Lymphoid precursors
D. Megakaryocytes

Q43. Which of the following stem cell sources is associated with a higher risk of graft-versus-host disease (GVHD) in allogeneic transplant?

A. Peripheral blood stem cells
B. Bone marrow
C. Umbilical cord blood
D. Autologous stem cells

Q44. Which preparative regimen is used to eliminate recipient hematopoietic cells prior to allogeneic transplant?

A. Myeloablative conditioning
B. Reduced-intensity conditioning
C. Graft-versus-host disease prophylaxis

D. Immunoglobulin therapy

Q45. Which condition is most likely to require a non-myeloablative preparative regimen?

A. Severe aplastic anemia
B. Acute myeloid leukemia in remission
C. Advanced multiple myeloma
D. Chronic lymphocytic leukemia

Q46. Which of the following is the primary goal of stem cell mobilization in preparation for autologous transplantation?

A. To reduce tumor burden
B. To increase the number of circulating stem cells for collection
C. To prevent infection during the transplant process
D. To eliminate recipient hematopoietic cells

Q47. Which is the most common method for collecting stem cells for autologous transplantation?

A. Apheresis from peripheral blood
B. Bone marrow aspiration
C. Umbilical cord blood collection
D. Stem cell biopsy

Q48. Which HLA class I molecule is most important in presenting antigens to CD8+ cytotoxic T cells?

A. HLA-A
B. HLA-B
C. HLA-DR
D. HLA-DQ

Q49. Which type of graft is associated with a higher risk of graft-versus-host disease (GVHD) in allogeneic transplant?

A. Autologous graft
B. Matched sibling graft
C. Unrelated donor graft
D. Umbilical cord blood graft

Q50. Which of the following is most closely associated with a higher risk of GVHD following an allogeneic stem cell transplant?

A. Older donor age
B. Female donor to male recipient
C. Female donor to female recipient
D. HLA match at 4/6 loci

Q51. Which cytokine plays a central role in stem cell mobilization from the bone marrow into peripheral blood?

A. Tumor necrosis factor-alpha
B. Granulocyte-colony stimulating factor (G-CSF)
C. Interleukin-1
D. Interferon-gamma

Q52. Which of the following is an indication for autologous stem cell transplantation?

A. Acute myeloid leukemia in remission
B. Chronic lymphocytic leukemia in remission
C. Multiple myeloma with refractory disease
D. Severe aplastic anemia

Q53. Which of the following cells is most responsible for the development of acute graft-versus-host disease (GVHD)?

A. Neutrophils

B. B lymphocytes
C. T lymphocytes
D. Macrophages

Q54. Which of the following is most likely to increase the risk of graft failure after transplant?
A. Graft-versus-host disease
B. Poor HLA match
C. Prolonged neutropenia
D. Chronic graft-versus-tumor effect

Q55. What is the primary purpose of using total body irradiation (TBI) in the preparative regimen for allogeneic stem cell transplantation?
A. To induce graft-versus-tumor effect
B. To eliminate host hematopoietic cells
C. To reduce the risk of infection
D. To enhance immune recovery

Q56. Which molecule is most commonly used to deplete T cells from a donor graft in an attempt to reduce graft-versus-host disease (GVHD)?
A. Anti-thymocyte globulin (ATG)
B. Rituximab
C. Cyclophosphamide
D. Etoposide

Q57. Which of the following conditions is most commonly associated with the development of chronic graft-versus-host disease (GVHD)?
A. Autologous stem cell transplant
B. Fully matched sibling donor transplant
C. Umbilical cord blood transplant
D. Mismatched unrelated donor transplant

Q58. Which cytokine is primarily responsible for immune reconstitution and preventing graft rejection after allogeneic hematopoietic stem cell transplantation?
A. Interferon-gamma
B. Interleukin-2 (IL-2)
C. Tumor necrosis factor-alpha (TNF-alpha)
D. Granulocyte-colony stimulating factor (G-CSF)

Q59. Which of the following is a common side effect of granulocyte-colony stimulating factor (G-CSF) used for stem cell mobilization?
A. Hair loss
B. Bone pain
C. Nausea
D. Skin rash

Q60. Which of the following is the primary purpose of using prophylactic antibiotics in the early post-transplant period?
A. To prevent GVHD
B. To enhance immune reconstitution
C. To prevent infections due to neutropenia
D. To promote stem cell engraftment

Q61. Which type of transplant involves the infusion of stem cells from the patient's own body?
A. Allogeneic transplant
B. Autologous transplant
C. Syngeneic transplant

D. Haploidentical transplant

Q62. Which of the following is a characteristic of myeloablative conditioning?

A. Suppression of host immune system without destroying host hematopoiesis
B. Total elimination of recipient hematopoietic cells
C. Non-toxic to donor stem cells
D. Limited use in older patients due to high toxicity

Q63. Which of the following is a significant complication of allogeneic stem cell transplantation?

A. Graft-versus-host disease (GVHD)
B. Hypertension
C. Thromboembolic events
D. Osteoarthritis

Q64. Which condition is most commonly treated with an allogeneic stem cell transplant?

A. Severe aplastic anemia
B. Multiple sclerosis
C. Alzheimer's disease
D. Osteoarthritis

Q65. Which of the following is the primary challenge when using umbilical cord blood for hematopoietic stem cell transplantation?

A. Limited T-cell count
B. Excessive risk of GVHD
C. High risk of graft rejection
D. Difficulty in HLA matching

Q66. Which cytokine is most commonly used to mobilize stem cells into peripheral blood for collection?

A. Interferon-gamma
B. Granulocyte-colony stimulating factor (G-CSF)
C. Tumor necrosis factor-alpha (TNF-alpha)
D. Interleukin-2 (IL-2)

Q67. Which of the following stem cell sources is most commonly used in allogeneic transplantation for adult patients?

A. Umbilical cord blood
B. Bone marrow
C. Peripheral blood stem cells
D. Placental blood

Q68. Which of the following pre-transplant tests is most important for assessing the risk of infection during the post-transplant period?

A. Echocardiogram
B. Pulmonary function tests
C. Chest x-ray
D. Serologic testing for viral infections (e.g., CMV, EBV)

Q69. Which of the following is a key feature of chronic graft-versus-host disease (GVHD)?

A. Hyperacute onset of skin rash and fever
B. Chronic inflammation and fibrosis of affected organs
C. Rapid resolution following immune suppression
D. Lack of organ involvement

Q70. Which of the following is a major cause of infection in the early post-transplant period?

A. Graft-versus-tumor effect
B. Neutropenia from chemotherapy and conditioning regimens

C. Graft-versus-host disease
D. Chronic immunosuppression

Q71. What is the mechanism of action of anti-thymocyte globulin (ATG) in preventing graft rejection?
A. Depleting donor T-cells to prevent GVHD
B. Suppressing donor-derived cytotoxic T cells to reduce graft rejection
C. Enhancing host immune reactivity to eliminate recipient tumor cells
D. Stimulating host immune cells to prevent graft failure

Q72. Which of the following is the most common source of stem cells in pediatric allogeneic transplants?
A. Bone marrow
B. Peripheral blood stem cells
C. Umbilical cord blood
D. Autologous stem cells

Q73. Which of the following best describes the role of T-cells in graft-versus-tumor (GvT) effect?
A. T-cells reject donor cells after transplantation
B. T-cells attack malignant cells in the recipient after transplant
C. T-cells prevent engraftment of donor cells
D. T-cells help recipient immune cells recover after transplant

Q74. Which of the following factors most significantly contributes to the success of cord blood transplantation in adults?
A. Higher stem cell content in cord blood
B. Reduced incidence of graft-versus-host disease (GVHD)
C. Simpler HLA matching process
D. Lower cost compared to bone marrow

Q75. What is the most important consideration when selecting a donor for an allogeneic transplant?
A. The recipient's gender
B. The degree of HLA matching
C. The donor's blood type
D. The donor's age

Q76. Which of the following strategies is most commonly used to reduce the risk of graft rejection in allogeneic transplantation?
A. Using autologous stem cells
B. HLA-matching between donor and recipient
C. Conditioning the donor with chemotherapy
D. Administering immunosuppressive therapy to the donor

Q77. What is the primary function of stem cell mobilization agents like G-CSF?
A. To increase the number of stem cells in the peripheral blood
B. To stimulate immune system recovery
C. To prevent graft-versus-host disease
D. To enhance graft-versus-tumor effect

Q78. Which of the following is most likely to occur in a patient who experiences graft-versus-host disease (GVHD) after allogeneic transplant?
A. Reduced graft failure risk
B. Increased infection risk due to immunosuppression
C. Increased engraftment efficiency
D. Faster recovery of hematopoiesis

Q79. Which of the following best describes the role of conditioning regimens in hematopoietic stem cell transplantation?

A. To eliminate recipient hematopoietic cells and allow for donor engraftment
B. To stimulate the recipient's immune system to fight off infections
C. To promote the proliferation of donor stem cells
D. To reduce the risk of graft-versus-host disease

Q80. What is the primary benefit of using peripheral blood stem cells (PBSC) over bone marrow for allogeneic transplantation?
A. Faster engraftment
B. Lower risk of graft-versus-host disease
C. Reduced need for donor immunosuppressive therapy
D. Increased donor cell number

Q81. Which cell type is primarily responsible for phagocytosis during the early post-transplant period?
A. T lymphocytes
B. B lymphocytes
C. Neutrophils
D. Erythrocytes

Q82. Which of the following is an advantage of using bone marrow as a stem cell source for allogeneic transplantation?
A. Easier to collect than peripheral blood
B. Lower risk of graft-versus-host disease
C. Higher rate of stem cell engraftment
D. Better immune reconstitution compared to cord blood

Q83. Which of the following is the primary function of granulocyte-colony stimulating factor (G-CSF) in stem cell mobilization?
A. Stimulate the production of platelets
B. Stimulate the production of red blood cells
C. Stimulate the production of white blood cells and mobilize stem cells into the peripheral blood
D. Suppress the immune response to prevent GVHD

Q84. What is the primary goal of using myeloablative conditioning in allogeneic hematopoietic stem cell transplantation?
A. To reduce the risk of graft-versus-host disease
B. To eliminate the recipient's hematopoietic cells and make space for the donor cells
C. To enhance the immune response of the recipient
D. To prevent graft failure and reduce infection risk

Q85. Which of the following best describes the role of T regulatory cells (Tregs) in allogeneic stem cell transplantation?
A. Tregs increase graft-versus-host disease by activating donor T cells
B. Tregs decrease graft-versus-host disease by suppressing immune responses
C. Tregs enhance graft-versus-tumor effect by stimulating immune cells
D. Tregs are not involved in allogeneic stem cell transplantation

Q86. Which of the following is the most likely cause of delayed engraftment in an allogeneic stem cell transplant recipient?
A. Higher HLA match between donor and recipient
B. Use of non-myeloablative conditioning regimen
C. Administration of high doses of immunosuppressive therapy
D. Early onset of graft-versus-host disease (GVHD)

Q87. Which donor source is most commonly associated with the lowest risk of graft-versus-host disease (GVHD)?
A. Peripheral blood stem cells

B. Bone marrow
C. Umbilical cord blood
D. Haploidentical donor

Q88. Which of the following is a common side effect of G-CSF during stem cell mobilization?
A. Hair loss
B. Bone pain
C. Nausea
D. Skin rash

Q89. Which of the following strategies is used to reduce the incidence of graft-versus-host disease (GVHD) in an allogeneic stem cell transplant?
A. Administering high doses of chemotherapy before transplant
B. Using immunosuppressive therapy to prevent T-cell activation
C. Selecting donors based on ABO compatibility
D. Using autologous stem cells instead of allogeneic

Q90. Which of the following is the primary goal of the graft-versus-tumor (GvT) effect in allogeneic hematopoietic stem cell transplantation?
A. To destroy the host's immune system
B. To induce immune reconstitution
C. To eradicate residual malignant cells in the recipient
D. To prevent graft failure

Q91. Which of the following stem cell sources has the highest risk of graft rejection?
A. Autologous stem cells
B. Bone marrow from a matched sibling
C. Umbilical cord blood
D. Unrelated donor peripheral blood stem cells

Q92. Which of the following complications is commonly associated with the use of peripheral blood stem cells (PBSC) for allogeneic transplantation?
A. Increased risk of graft-versus-host disease (GVHD)
B. Lower risk of infection
C. Faster engraftment compared to bone marrow
D. Increased risk of graft rejection

Q93. Which cytokine plays a central role in the graft-versus-tumor (GvT) effect?
A. Interleukin-2 (IL-2)
B. Granulocyte-colony stimulating factor (G-CSF)
C. Tumor necrosis factor-alpha (TNF-alpha)
D. Interferon-gamma (IFN-gamma)

Q94. Which factor most influences the speed of stem cell engraftment in allogeneic transplantation?
A. Donor age
B. Conditioning regimen intensity
C. Donor gender
D. HLA match between donor and recipient

Q95. Which of the following complications is most commonly associated with umbilical cord blood transplantation?
A. Graft-versus-host disease (GVHD)
B. Engraftment delay
C. Infection risk
D. Chronic graft-versus-host disease (GVHD)

Q96. What is the major purpose of using anti-thymocyte globulin (ATG) in the pre-transplant regimen?

A. To deplete recipient T cells and prevent rejection
B. To prevent infection during the transplant process
C. To enhance stem cell engraftment
D. To stimulate immune response against malignant cells

Q97. Which of the following best describes the function of T-helper cells during an allogeneic stem cell transplant?

A. They activate B cells to produce antibodies
B. They destroy recipient tissue during graft-versus-host disease (GVHD)
C. They help activate cytotoxic T cells to fight tumor cells
D. They suppress immune responses to donor cells

Q98. Which of the following is most commonly used to treat GVHD in allogeneic transplant recipients?

A. Antiviral agents
B. Immunosuppressive drugs (e.g., corticosteroids)
C. Antibiotics
D. Growth factors

Q99. Which of the following immunosuppressive agents is commonly used for preventing graft-versus-host disease (GVHD) after allogeneic transplantation?

A. Methotrexate
B. Tacrolimus
C. Etoposide
D. Cyclophosphamide

Q100. Which of the following is a characteristic feature of umbilical cord blood stem cells?

A. Higher HLA matching requirement than peripheral blood
B. Increased risk of GVHD compared to bone marrow
C. Lower stem cell content compared to adult peripheral blood
D. Faster engraftment compared to bone marrow

Answer key and Explanation (1-100)
Q1. Answer: B
Explanation: Peripheral blood stem cells are the most commonly used source for autologous transplants due to faster engraftment. Option A – bone marrow is less commonly used autologously today. Option C – cord blood is rarely used for autologous adult transplants. Option D – placental stem cells are not a standard source.
SubChapter: D. Sources of stem cells
Q2. Answer: C
Explanation: HLA-A is a class I HLA molecule that presents peptides to CD8+ T cells. Option A – HLA-DR is class II and presents to CD4+ T cells. Option B – HLA-DQ is class II, not class I. Option D – HLA-DP is class II, not class I.
SubChapter: A. Basic concepts of transplantation — Histocompatibility
Q3. Answer: B
Explanation: A fully HLA-matched sibling is a matched related donor. Option A – MURD is unrelated, not sibling. Option C – haploidentical denotes a half-match, not full match. Option D – mismatched unrelated donor is not fully matched.
SubChapter: C. Types of transplants — Allogeneic (matched related donors)
Q4. Answer: B
Explanation: The graft-versus-tumor effect is an immune-mediated antitumor action that supports long-term disease control. Option A – neutrophil recovery reduces infection risk but not long-term tumor control. Option C – transfusion independence is supportive care, not tumor control. Option D – preventing mucositis addresses symptoms, not malignancy eradication.
SubChapter: A. Cellular goals of therapy (graft-versus-tumor effect)
Q5. Answer: A
Explanation: Flow cytometry enumerates CD34+ cells in blood and guides timing and adequacy of collection. Option B – CBC gives counts but not CD34 enumeration. Option C – ferritin assesses iron stores, not stem cells. Option D – cultures detect infection, not progenitor counts.
SubChapter: D. Sources of stem cells — Peripheral blood
Q6. Answer: B
Explanation: Severe aplastic anemia refractory to therapy is a standard indication for transplant. Option A – localized prostate cancer is not a transplant indication. Option C – iron deficiency is treated medically. Option D – osteoarthritis is not an indication.
SubChapter: B. Hematologic indications for transplantation
Q7. Answer: B
Explanation: The World Marrow Donor Association (WMDA) coordinates international donor registries and standards. Option A – CIBMTR collects outcomes data, not donor registries. Option C – ASBMT is a professional society, not the global donor registry. Option D – NCI is a research institute, not a donor registry operator.
SubChapter: H. Donor selection, care, and education
Q8. Answer: D
Explanation: Non-myeloablative regimens reduce intensity, focusing on immune suppression to permit donor chimerism. Option A – myeloablative destroys host marrow. Option C – hematopoietic rescue refers to reinfusion, not regimen intensity. Option B – total marrow ablation is equivalent to high-intensity myeloablation.
SubChapter: C. Conditioning / preparative regimens — Intensity of therapy
Q9. Answer: B

Explanation: Erythrocytes derive from the myeloid lineage (common myeloid progenitor). Option A – T cells derive from lymphoid progenitors. Option C – B cells derive from lymphoid lineage. Option D – NK cells are lymphoid lineage.
SubChapter: A. Hematopoietic cell lineage and function
Q10. Answer: B
Explanation: Peripheral blood stem cell grafts are associated with higher chronic GVHD rates compared with bone marrow or cord blood. Option A – cord blood has lower GVHD risk. Option C – autologous grafts do not cause GVHD. Option D – platelet transfusions are irrelevant to GVHD.
SubChapter: C. Types of transplants — Peripheral blood risk
Q11. Answer: A
Explanation: Uncontrolled severe heart failure is typically a contraindication until medically optimized because of high regimen-related risk. Option B – cardiac status is essential. Option C – heart failure worsens outcomes. Option D – heart failure affects peri-transplant risk and eligibility.
SubChapter: E. Recipient suitability and evaluation
Q12. Answer: B
Explanation: Cord blood contains immunologically naïve cells with reduced alloreactivity, allowing greater HLA mismatch tolerance. Option A – cord blood often has lower CD34+ dose in adults. Option C – cord blood lacks robust adult memory T cells. Option D – cord blood does not guarantee permanent adult donor chimerism more than other sources.
SubChapter: D. Sources of stem cells — Umbilical cord
Q13. Answer: B
Explanation: Infection prevention and warning signs to contact the team are critical discharge education topics. Option A – genomic methods are not immediate discharge priorities. Option C – radiotherapy techniques are rarely relevant to patient self-care. Option D – instrument calibration is irrelevant to patient education.
SubChapter: F. Recipient education
Q14. Answer: B
Explanation: Complement pathways and neutrophils mediate early defense against encapsulated bacteria. Option A – CD8+ T cells are key for viral/intracellular defense. Option C – stromal cells support marrow but not immediate antibacterial defense. Option D – erythrocytes transport oxygen, not immune defense.
SubChapter: A. Immune system and function
Q15. Answer: C
Explanation: Higher donor T-cell content correlates with increased GVHD risk. Option A – ABO mismatch typically affects hemolytic issues but not GVHD risk markedly. Option B – donor parity (e.g., multiparous female) can increase GVHD risk, so parity is relevant. Option D – donor younger than recipient does not universally reduce GVHD risk.
SubChapter: H. Donor selection, care, and education — graft composition
Q16. Answer: B
Explanation: Serology for CMV, EBV, and hepatitis viruses evaluates latent infectious risk pre-transplant. Option A – PFTs assess lung function, not viral status. Option C – echo assesses cardiac risk. Option D – bone density assesses fracture risk, not infection.
SubChapter: E. Recipient suitability and evaluation — infection risk
Q17. Answer: A
Explanation: Chimerism testing quantifies donor/recipient cell proportions to evaluate engraftment and risk of rejection/relapse. Option B – cytokines are different assays. Option C – chimerism can be clinically useful. Option D – chimerism is unrelated to renal function assessment.
SubChapter: III.F (noted in Outline) — Chimerism (but foundational concept: engraftment monitoring)

Q18. Answer: A
Explanation: High-dose alkylating agents commonly cause mucosal barrier injury and mucositis. Option B – antihistamines do not cause mucositis. Option C – emollients are supportive care, not causative. Option D – intranasal vaccines are unrelated.
SubChapter: II.C. Conditioning / preparative regimens — Chemotherapy
Q19. Answer: B
Explanation: Both patient and primary caregiver(s) should receive education on infection precautions and care responsibilities. Option A – excluding caregivers omits essential support. Option C – spectators do not need clinical caregiving instruction. Option D – the team already knows these topics; education is for patient/caregiver.
SubChapter: G. Caregiver education
Q20. Answer: A
Explanation: CAR-T is a cellular immunotherapy distinct from classic HSC grafts and is listed under cellular therapies. Option B – azithromycin is an antimicrobial, not cellular therapy. Option C – topical steroids are supportive care. Option D – vaccinations are preventive, not cellular therapies.
SubChapter: II.F. Cellular therapies (e.g., CAR-T)
Q21. Answer: B
Explanation: The kidney secretes erythropoietin to stimulate erythrocyte production during hypoxia. Option A – the liver contributes mainly in fetal life. Option C – the spleen filters blood, not hormone production. Option D – marrow responds to, not produces, EPO.
SubChapter: A. Hematopoietic cell lineage and function
Q22. Answer: A
Explanation: Donor CD8$^+$ T cells recognize host HLA antigens and mediate GVHD. Option B – neutrophils fight infection, not GVHD. Option C – platelets have no immune recognition. Option D – erythrocytes lack nuclei, not immune cells.
SubChapter: A. Immune system and function
Q23. Answer: C
Explanation: COPD is not a hematologic indication for transplant. Option A – AML is classic indication. Option B – autologous HSCT used in myeloma. Option D – standard for severe aplastic anemia.
SubChapter: B. Hematologic indications for transplantation
Q24. Answer: C
Explanation: Haploidentical pairs share one parental haplotype (≈50% match). Option A – identical is full match. Option B – fully mismatched not haploidentical. Option D – ABO grouping is separate from HLA.
SubChapter: C. Types of transplants — haploidentical
Q25. Answer: B
Explanation: CD4$^+$ cells coordinate adaptive immunity and stimulate B cells. Option A – EPO from kidney. Option C – phagocytosis done by macrophages/neutrophils. Option D – platelets handle aggregation.
SubChapter: A. Immune system and function
Q26. Answer: B
Explanation: HLA typing is the key criterion for related donor eligibility. Option A – ABO is secondary. Option C – recipient labs don't select donor. Option D – age affects outcome but not primary selection.
SubChapter: H. Donor selection, care and education
Q27. Answer: C
Explanation: CD34 marks early hematopoietic progenitors used for collection targeting. Option A – CD4 marks T helpers. Option B – CD8 cytotoxic T cells. Option D – CD19 B cells.
SubChapter: A. Hematopoietic cell lineage and function
Q28. Answer: B

Explanation: PBSC collection yields rapid engraftment and shorter cytopenia. Option A – storage methods similar. Option C – PBSC has higher $CD34^+$ count. Option D – mobilization adds cost.
SubChapter: D. Sources of stem cells
Q29. Answer: C
Explanation: Donor lymphocytes attack residual malignant cells (GvT effect). Option A – central tolerance prevents autoimmunity. Option B – anergy is non-responsiveness. Option D – peripheral tolerance limits auto-reactivity.
SubChapter: A. Cellular goals of therapy
Q30. Answer: B
Explanation: G-CSF stimulates stem cells to circulate for collection. Option A – it enhances release, not inhibit. Option C – does not kill cells. Option D – secondary mechanism but main action is mobilization.
SubChapter: D. Stem cell mobilization
Q31. Answer: A
Explanation: Donors must understand collection process and side effects. Option B – patient privacy. Option C – billing not relevant. Option D – recipient-focused.
SubChapter: H. Donor selection, care and education
Q32. Answer: C
Explanation: HLA-DR presents antigen to $CD4^+$ T cells. Option A/B/C – A and B are class I; C – class I too. DR is class II.
SubChapter: A. Histocompatibility
Q33. Answer: C
Explanation: Cord blood units are banked frozen until needed. Option A – fresh BM used immediately. Option B – often fresh or short-term frozen. Option D – usually fresh.
SubChapter: D. Sources of stem cells — cord blood
Q34. Answer: A
Explanation: Marrow involvement risks reinfusing malignant cells. Option B – accepted autologous indication. Option C – standard autologous use. Option D – salvage setting OK.
SubChapter: B. Indications for transplantation
Q35. Answer: A
Explanation: Engraftment is successful donor cell proliferation in recipient marrow. Option B – cell death. Option C – granule release. Option D – clot breakdown.
SubChapter: A. Cellular goals of therapy — hematologic reconstitution
Q36. Answer: D
Explanation: PFTs assess baseline lung capacity for chemoradiation tolerance. Option B – abdominal imaging unrelated. Option C/A – not used for conditioning assessment.
SubChapter: E. Recipient suitability and evaluation
Q37. Answer: A
Explanation: Engraftment is achieved when ANC > 500 for 3 days. Option B – defines platelet recovery. Option C – too low for engraftment. Option D – collection target, not engraftment.
SubChapter: A. Hematologic reconstitution
Q38. Answer: A
Explanation: Hydration and calcium monitoring prevent citrate toxicity and complications. Option B – not educational priority. Option C/D – technical or administrative.
SubChapter: H. Donor education
Q39. Answer: B
Explanation: Platelets form from megakaryocyte cytoplasmic fragments. Option A – myeloblasts → granulocytes. Option C/D – not precursors to platelets.
SubChapter: A. Hematopoietic cell lineage and function

Q40. Answer: A
Explanation: CAR-T uses patient's T cells engineered to attack tumor antigens. Option B – no chemotherapy alone. Option C – not stem cell based. Option D – used in B-cell malignancies.
SubChapter: II.F Cellular therapies (CAR-T)
Q41. Answer: B
Explanation: HLA typing is the gold standard for assessing donor-recipient compatibility. Option A – glucose levels are unrelated. Option C – blood culture identifies infection, not compatibility. Option D – biopsy evaluates marrow health, not compatibility.
SubChapter: A. Histocompatibility
Q42. Answer: D
Explanation: Megakaryocytes are the precursor cells that produce platelets. Option A – erythroid cells produce red blood cells. Option B – myeloid precursors produce granulocytes and monocytes. Option C – lymphoid precursors produce T and B cells.
SubChapter: A. Hematopoietic cell lineage and function
Q43. Answer: A
Explanation: Peripheral blood stem cells contain more T cells, which increase the risk of GVHD. Option B – bone marrow is associated with a lower risk of GVHD. Option C – cord blood has a lower T-cell count, reducing GVHD risk. Option D – autologous grafts do not cause GVHD.
SubChapter: C. Types of transplants
Q44. Answer: A
Explanation: Myeloablative conditioning eliminates recipient marrow to allow donor engraftment. Option B – reduced intensity targets immune suppression, not complete myeloablation. Option C – GVHD prophylaxis is a separate strategy. Option D – immunoglobulin therapy helps prevent infections, not conditioning.
SubChapter: C. Conditioning / preparative regimens
Q45. Answer: D
Explanation: Non-myeloablative regimens are often used in CLL due to the disease's slower progression. Option A – myeloablative therapy is more common for aplastic anemia. Option B – AML in remission typically requires myeloablative conditioning. Option C – myeloblative therapy is standard for myeloma.
SubChapter: C. Conditioning / preparative regimens
Q46. Answer: B
Explanation: Mobilization increases circulating stem cells for collection. Option A – mobilization does not directly reduce tumor burden. Option C – infection prevention is post-transplant care. Option D – this occurs with preparative regimens, not mobilization.
SubChapter: D. Stem cell mobilization
Q47. Answer: A
Explanation: Apheresis is the most common method for collecting stem cells in autologous transplants. Option B – bone marrow aspiration is used in fewer cases. Option C – cord blood is not commonly used for adults. Option D – stem cell biopsy does not exist.
SubChapter: D. Sources of stem cells
Q48. Answer: A
Explanation: HLA-A molecules present antigens to CD8+ T cells. Option B – HLA-B also presents to CD8+, but HLA-A is most studied. Option C – HLA-DR presents to CD4+ T cells. Option D – HLA-DQ is class II, presenting to CD4+ T cells.
SubChapter: A. Histocompatibility
Q49. Answer: C

Explanation: Unrelated donor grafts carry a higher GVHD risk due to T-cell mismatch. Option A – autologous grafts cannot cause GVHD. Option B – matched sibling grafts are less likely to cause GVHD. Option D – cord blood has fewer T cells, reducing GVHD risk.
SubChapter: C. Types of transplants

Q50. Answer: B

Explanation: Female donors to male recipients are more likely to develop GVHD due to maternal immune memory. Option A – donor age can affect outcomes but is less relevant to GVHD. Option C – GVHD risk is higher with male recipients. Option D – incomplete HLA matching increases GVHD risk.
SubChapter: H. Donor selection, care and education

Q51. Answer: B

Explanation: G-CSF stimulates stem cell mobilization from marrow into peripheral blood. Option A – TNF-alpha is involved in inflammation, not mobilization. Option C – IL-1 is pro-inflammatory but not involved in mobilization. Option D – interferon-gamma is involved in immune responses, not mobilization.
SubChapter: D. Stem cell mobilization

Q52. Answer: C

Explanation: Autologous stem cell transplant is used in multiple myeloma to restore hematopoiesis after chemotherapy. Option A – myeloid leukemia often requires allogeneic transplant. Option B – CLL usually treated with non-transplant therapies. Option D – aplastic anemia requires allogeneic transplant.
SubChapter: B. Hematologic indications for transplantation

Q53. Answer: C

Explanation: T lymphocytes from the donor attack recipient tissues, causing acute GVHD. Option A – neutrophils mediate infection response, not GVHD. Option B – B lymphocytes are involved in humoral immunity, not GVHD. Option D – macrophages mediate inflammation but not GVHD.
SubChapter: A. Immune system and function

Q54. Answer: B

Explanation: Poor HLA matching increases graft failure risk due to immune rejection. Option A – GVHD affects host tissue, not graft failure. Option C – neutropenia delays recovery but doesn't directly cause graft failure. Option D – graft-versus-tumor helps eradicate malignancy, not graft function.
SubChapter: A. Cellular goals of therapy

Q55. Answer: B

Explanation: TBI eliminates host marrow to prepare for donor cell engraftment. Option A – graft-versus-tumor is mediated by donor T cells, not TBI. Option C – infection prevention is not TBI's primary goal. Option D – immune recovery follows after conditioning.
SubChapter: C. Conditioning / preparative regimens

Q56. Answer: A

Explanation: ATG is used to deplete T cells to reduce GVHD risk. Option B – rituximab targets B cells, not T cells. Option C – cyclophosphamide is a chemotherapy agent, not a T-cell depletion agent. Option D – etoposide is used for conditioning, not T-cell depletion.
SubChapter: H. Donor selection, care and education

Q57. Answer: D

Explanation: Mismatched unrelated donor transplants have a higher risk of chronic GVHD. Option A – autologous grafts cannot cause GVHD. Option B – fully matched sibling grafts have lower GVHD risk. Option C – cord blood grafts have fewer T cells, lowering GVHD risk.
SubChapter: D. Sources of stem cells

Q58. Answer: B

Explanation: IL-2 is critical for T-cell expansion and immune reconstitution. Option A – interferon-gamma is involved in immune responses but not reconstitution. Option C – TNF-alpha is involved in

inflammation, not immune reconstitution. Option D – G-CSF supports neutrophil recovery, not T-cell reconstitution.
SubChapter: A. Immune system and function

Q59. Answer: B

Explanation: Bone pain is a common side effect of G-CSF due to increased stem cell mobilization. Option A – hair loss is more common with chemotherapy. Option C – nausea is rare with G-CSF. Option D – skin rash is not a typical G-CSF side effect.
SubChapter: D. Stem cell mobilization

Q60. Answer: C

Explanation: Prophylactic antibiotics prevent infections in the neutropenic phase. Option A – antibiotics do not prevent GVHD. Option B – immune reconstitution occurs naturally over time. Option D – antibiotics support infection prevention, not engraftment.
SubChapter: III. Infection prevention and management

Q61. Answer: B

Explanation: An autologous transplant uses the patient's own stem cells. Option A – allogeneic uses stem cells from a donor. Option C – syngeneic uses stem cells from an identical twin. Option D – haploidentical uses stem cells from a half-matched relative.
SubChapter: C. Types of transplants

Q62. Answer: B

Explanation: Myeloablative conditioning fully eliminates recipient hematopoietic cells to make room for donor stem cells. Option A – immune suppression occurs but doesn't eliminate hematopoiesis. Option C – conditioning doesn't target donor cells. Option D – it's typically too toxic for older patients.
SubChapter: C. Conditioning / preparative regimens

Q63. Answer: A

Explanation: GVHD is a major complication in allogeneic transplants, where the donor immune cells attack the recipient's tissues. Option B – hypertension is common but not specific to transplant. Option C – thromboembolic events occur but are not primary complications. Option D – osteoarthritis is unrelated.
SubChapter: A. Cellular goals of therapy

Q64. Answer: A

Explanation: Allogeneic stem cell transplantation is used for hematologic disorders like severe aplastic anemia. Option B – multiple sclerosis may be treated with immunotherapies, not stem cells. Option C – Alzheimer's disease is not treated with stem cell transplants. Option D – osteoarthritis is unrelated to stem cell transplantation.
SubChapter: B. Hematologic indications for transplantation

Q65. Answer: A

Explanation: Umbilical cord blood has a lower T-cell count, which reduces GVHD but limits immune reconstitution. Option B – lower T-cells actually reduce GVHD. Option C – graft rejection is lower in cord blood. Option D – cord blood typically involves a less stringent HLA match.
SubChapter: D. Sources of stem cells — Umbilical cord blood

Q66. Answer: B

Explanation: G-CSF is used to mobilize stem cells into peripheral blood for collection. Option A – interferon-gamma enhances immune responses, not mobilization. Option C – TNF-alpha is inflammatory, not for mobilization. Option D – IL-2 stimulates T-cell growth, not stem cell mobilization.
SubChapter: D. Stem cell mobilization

Q67. Answer: C

Explanation: Peripheral blood stem cells are the most commonly used for allogeneic adult transplants due to better engraftment rates. Option A – cord blood is often reserved for pediatric use. Option B – bone marrow is still used but less frequently. Option D – placental blood is not commonly used in adults.
SubChapter: D. Sources of stem cells

Q68. Answer: D

Explanation: Serologic testing for viral infections is crucial for assessing infection risk in transplant patients. Option A – echocardiogram assesses heart function, not infection risk. Option B – pulmonary tests assess lung function, not infection. Option C – chest x-ray may detect pneumonia but not viral risk.
SubChapter: E. Recipient suitability and evaluation

Q69. Answer: B

Explanation: Chronic GVHD involves long-term inflammation and fibrosis of organs like skin, liver, and gastrointestinal tract. Option A – hyperacute GVHD occurs acutely, not chronically. Option C – chronic GVHD typically requires prolonged treatment. Option D – chronic GVHD involves multiple organs.
SubChapter: A. Immune system and function

Q70. Answer: B

Explanation: Neutropenia from chemotherapy and conditioning regimens significantly increases the risk of infection in the early post-transplant period. Option A – GvT effect targets malignancy, not infection. Option C – GVHD is a later complication. Option D – chronic immunosuppression is more relevant later.
SubChapter: III. Infection prevention and management

Q71. Answer: B

Explanation: ATG depletes donor T-cells, reducing the risk of graft rejection. Option A – ATG is used for T-cell depletion, not GVHD prevention. Option C – ATG does not stimulate immune reactivity. Option D – ATG suppresses immune response, not stimulates it.
SubChapter: H. Donor selection, care and education

Q72. Answer: C

Explanation: Umbilical cord blood is commonly used in pediatric transplants due to better immune tolerance. Option A – bone marrow is less commonly used in children. Option B – peripheral blood is more common in adults. Option D – autologous grafts are not used in allogeneic transplants.
SubChapter: D. Sources of stem cells

Q73. Answer: B

Explanation: T-cells mediate the graft-versus-tumor effect by attacking residual malignant cells. Option A – T-cells reject grafts in GVHD, not GvT. Option C – T-cells facilitate engraftment, not rejection. Option D – T-cells support anti-tumor responses, not immune recovery.
SubChapter: A. Cellular goals of therapy

Q74. Answer: B

Explanation: Cord blood has a lower incidence of GVHD due to fewer T-cells. Option A – cord blood has lower stem cell content than peripheral blood. Option C – HLA matching is often more complex with cord blood. Option D – cost is not a primary advantage of cord blood.
SubChapter: D. Sources of stem cells

Q75. Answer: B

Explanation: The degree of HLA matching is the most important factor in reducing the risk of graft rejection. Option A – gender is less important than HLA match. Option C – blood type compatibility is secondary. Option D – age affects outcomes but not primary compatibility.
SubChapter: H. Donor selection, care and education

Q76. Answer: B

Explanation: HLA-matching is the key to reducing the risk of graft rejection. Option A – autologous transplants avoid rejection risk. Option C – conditioning affects the recipient, not the donor. Option D – immunosuppressive therapy is given to the recipient.

SubChapter: H. Donor selection, care and education

Q77. Answer: A

Explanation: G-CSF increases the number of stem cells in the peripheral blood for collection. Option B – G-CSF does not stimulate immune recovery. Option C – G-CSF does not prevent GVHD. Option D – G-CSF is not involved in GvT.

SubChapter: D. Stem cell mobilization

Q78. Answer: B

Explanation: GVHD involves immune-mediated damage and increases infection risk due to required immunosuppression. Option A – GVHD increases rejection risk. Option C – GVHD complicates, not enhances, engraftment. Option D – GVHD impairs recovery and delays hematopoiesis.

SubChapter: A. Cellular goals of therapy

Q79. Answer: A

Explanation: Conditioning regimens eliminate recipient cells to allow donor cells to engraft. Option B – immune stimulation is not the main role of conditioning. Option C – conditioning doesn't promote donor stem cells, it clears space. Option D – conditioning does not directly reduce GVHD.

SubChapter: C. Conditioning / preparative regimens

Q80. Answer: A

Explanation: PBSC transplants lead to faster engraftment compared to bone marrow. Option B – PBSC can increase GVHD risk due to higher T-cell content. Option C – both PBSC and bone marrow require immunosuppression. Option D – marrow often yields more stem cells per donor.

SubChapter: D. Sources of stem cells

Q81. Answer: C

Explanation: Neutrophils are the primary phagocytes during the early post-transplant period. Option A – T lymphocytes are key for immune regulation, not phagocytosis. Option B – B lymphocytes produce antibodies but do not phagocytize. Option D – erythrocytes transport oxygen, not pathogens.

SubChapter: A. Immune system and function

Q82. Answer: B

Explanation: Bone marrow has a lower risk of graft-versus-host disease due to fewer T cells compared to peripheral blood. Option A – peripheral blood is easier to collect. Option C – PBSC has higher engraftment rates. Option D – cord blood has less immune reconstitution, not bone marrow.

SubChapter: D. Sources of stem cells

Q83. Answer: C

Explanation: G-CSF stimulates white blood cell production and mobilizes stem cells from the bone marrow into peripheral blood. Option A – platelets are produced by megakaryocytes, not G-CSF. Option B – red blood cells are produced by erythropoietin. Option D – G-CSF does not prevent GVHD.

SubChapter: D. Stem cell mobilization

Q84. Answer: B

Explanation: Myeloablative conditioning eliminates recipient hematopoietic cells to allow for donor engraftment. Option A – GVHD prevention is addressed by immunosuppressive agents, not conditioning. Option C – conditioning suppresses the immune system. Option D – conditioning does not directly prevent graft failure, but helps engraftment.

SubChapter: C. Conditioning / preparative regimens

Q85. Answer: B

Explanation: Tregs suppress immune responses, helping to reduce GVHD in allogeneic transplants. Option A – Tregs inhibit immune responses, not activate them. Option C – Tregs do not enhance the GvT effect directly. Option D – Tregs play a key role in immune regulation.

SubChapter: A. Immune system and function

Q86. Answer: D

Explanation: GVHD can delay engraftment by damaging the newly transplanted stem cells. Option A – better HLA matching typically leads to faster engraftment. Option B – non-myeloablative regimens can cause slower engraftment but are not typically the primary cause. Option C – immunosuppressive therapy can delay engraftment, but GVHD has a larger impact.
SubChapter: A. Cellular goals of therapy

Q87. Answer: C

Explanation: Umbilical cord blood has fewer T cells, which significantly reduces the risk of GVHD. Option A – peripheral blood stem cells contain higher T cell counts, increasing GVHD risk. Option B – bone marrow also has fewer T cells, but less than cord blood. Option D – haploidentical transplants have a higher risk of GVHD.
SubChapter: D. Sources of stem cells

Q88. Answer: B

Explanation: Bone pain is a common side effect of G-CSF due to bone marrow stimulation. Option A – hair loss is associated with chemotherapy, not G-CSF. Option C – nausea is not a primary side effect of G-CSF. Option D – skin rash is uncommon with G-CSF.
SubChapter: D. Stem cell mobilization

Q89. Answer: B

Explanation: Immunosuppressive therapy is used to prevent T-cell activation, which reduces GVHD. Option A – high chemotherapy doses can damage stem cells, not prevent GVHD. Option C – ABO compatibility is secondary to HLA matching for GVHD prevention. Option D – autologous transplants do not cause GVHD.
SubChapter: A. Cellular goals of therapy

Q90. Answer: C

Explanation: GvT effect involves donor immune cells attacking and eradicating residual malignant cells. Option A – GvT doesn't target the host immune system, only the tumor. Option B – immune reconstitution occurs over time after transplant. Option D – graft failure is prevented by other factors, not GvT.
SubChapter: A. Cellular goals of therapy

Q91. Answer: D

Explanation: Unrelated donor peripheral blood stem cells have the highest risk of rejection due to immunologic differences. Option A – autologous grafts cannot be rejected. Option B – sibling bone marrow is most compatible. Option C – cord blood has a lower risk of rejection but other challenges.
SubChapter: C. Types of transplants

Q92. Answer: A

Explanation: PBSCs contain more T cells, which increases the risk of GVHD. Option B – PBSCs do not reduce infection risk. Option C – PBSCs generally lead to faster engraftment. Option D – PBSCs typically reduce graft rejection risk compared to mismatched grafts.
SubChapter: D. Sources of stem cells

Q93. Answer: D

Explanation: IFN-gamma plays a central role in the GvT effect by activating cytotoxic T cells. Option A – IL-2 promotes T cell proliferation, not GvT. Option B – G-CSF is used for stem cell mobilization, not GvT. Option C – TNF-alpha is involved in inflammation but not GvT.
SubChapter: A. Immune system and function

Q94. Answer: D

Explanation: The HLA match between donor and recipient is the most critical factor in the speed of engraftment. Option A – donor age can influence graft outcomes, but HLA match is more important. Option B – conditioning regimen intensity affects engraftment but not as much as HLA match. Option C – gender affects graft rejection but not engraftment speed.

SubChapter: A. Cellular goals of therapy

Q95. Answer: B

Explanation: Umbilical cord blood transplantation is associated with engraftment delay due to lower cell numbers. Option A – cord blood has a lower incidence of GVHD. Option C – infection risk is a general post-transplant concern, not specific to cord blood. Option D – GVHD risk is lower with cord blood.

SubChapter: D. Sources of stem cells

Q96. Answer: A

Explanation: ATG depletes recipient T cells to reduce the risk of rejection. Option B – ATG is not used to prevent infections. Option C – ATG does not enhance engraftment. Option D – ATG suppresses, not stimulates, the immune response.

SubChapter: H. Donor selection, care and education

Q97. Answer: C

Explanation: T-helper cells help activate cytotoxic T cells to target and eliminate tumor cells. Option A – B cell activation is not their main role in GvT. Option B – cytotoxic T cells, not T-helper cells, mediate GVHD. Option D – T-helper cells support immune responses, not suppress them.

SubChapter: A. Immune system and function

Q98. Answer: B

Explanation: Immunosuppressive drugs like corticosteroids are used to treat GVHD. Option A – antiviral agents treat infections, not GVHD. Option C – antibiotics prevent infections, not treat GVHD. Option D – growth factors aid engraftment, not GVHD management.

SubChapter: A. Cellular goals of therapy

Q99. Answer: B

Explanation: Tacrolimus is an immunosuppressive agent commonly used to prevent GVHD. Option A – methotrexate is used in combination with other drugs for GVHD prevention. Option C – etoposide is used in conditioning, not GVHD prevention. Option D – cyclophosphamide is used in conditioning regimens.

SubChapter: A. Immune system and function

Q100. Answer: C

Explanation: Umbilical cord blood has lower stem cell content compared to adult peripheral blood. Option A – cord blood often has a more relaxed HLA matching requirement. Option B – cord blood has a lower risk of GVHD. Option D – engraftment is typically slower with cord blood.

SubChapter: D. Sources of stem cells

Questions (101-200)

Q101. Which of the following is a key benefit of using umbilical cord blood as a stem cell source for transplantation?

A. Higher cell dose than peripheral blood
B. Lower risk of graft-versus-host disease (GVHD)
C. Faster engraftment compared to bone marrow
D. Greater HLA match requirement

Q102. Which aspect of hematopoietic stem cell transplant (HSCT) is most influenced by the donor's HLA compatibility with the recipient?

A. The risk of infection
B. The rate of graft rejection
C. The development of graft-versus-host disease (GVHD)
D. The speed of engraftment

Q103. Which of the following pre-transplant screening tests is critical for assessing latent viral infections in transplant candidates?

A. Bone marrow biopsy
B. Serologic testing for Epstein-Barr virus (EBV) and cytomegalovirus (CMV)
C. Pulmonary function tests
D. Echocardiogram

Q104. Which of the following is the primary reason for using total body irradiation (TBI) as part of the preparative regimen in allogeneic stem cell transplantation?

A. To prevent graft-versus-host disease (GVHD)
B. To kill tumor cells and suppress the immune system
C. To enhance stem cell engraftment
D. To eliminate the recipient's hematopoietic cells and make space for donor cells

Q105. In haploidentical stem cell transplantation, what is the primary challenge that affects outcomes?

A. Limited stem cell availability
B. High risk of graft-versus-host disease (GVHD)
C. Difficulty in HLA matching
D. Delayed immune reconstitution

Q106. Which cell population is most directly responsible for initiating graft-versus-host disease (GVHD) in allogeneic transplant recipients?

A. B lymphocytes
B. Neutrophils
C. T lymphocytes
D. Monocytes

Q107. What is the most common complication associated with stem cell mobilization in preparation for autologous transplant?

A. Graft rejection
B. Increased infection risk due to neutropenia
C. Bone pain from G-CSF administration
D. Liver toxicity

Q108. Which of the following is a benefit of using autologous stem cells for transplantation?

A. Elimination of the risk of graft-versus-host disease (GVHD)
B. Higher rate of engraftment than allogeneic grafts
C. Reduced risk of infection

D. Increased immune tolerance

Q109. What is the most common cause of early graft failure in allogeneic stem cell transplantation?

A. Graft-versus-host disease (GVHD)
B. Infection due to immunosuppression
C. Poor HLA matching
D. Delayed immune reconstitution

Q110. Which of the following is the primary mechanism by which cyclophosphamide prevents graft rejection in allogeneic transplants?

A. Depletion of host immune cells
B. Activation of donor immune cells to attack tumors
C. Enhancement of donor stem cell engraftment
D. Reduction of T-cell proliferation in the recipient

Q111. Which of the following is the primary role of T-cells in allogeneic hematopoietic stem cell transplantation?

A. To regulate graft-versus-host disease (GVHD)
B. To prevent infection after transplant
C. To mediate the graft-versus-tumor effect
D. To enhance the immune reconstitution

Q112. Which of the following is the most common cause of death in the early post-transplant period?

A. Graft rejection
B. Infection
C. Graft-versus-host disease (GVHD)
D. Malignant relapse

Q113. What is the primary function of anti-thymocyte globulin (ATG) in hematopoietic stem cell transplantation?

A. To stimulate immune reconstitution
B. To deplete recipient T-cells and prevent graft rejection
C. To enhance the graft-versus-tumor effect
D. To reduce the risk of infection

Q114. Which of the following is the most common complication of peripheral blood stem cell (PBSC) collection?

A. Bone pain
B. Anemia
C. Platelet deficiency
D. Graft-versus-host disease (GVHD)

Q115. Which stem cell source has the highest risk of graft rejection due to HLA mismatch?

A. Autologous stem cells
B. Bone marrow from a matched sibling
C. Umbilical cord blood
D. Unrelated donor peripheral blood stem cells

Q116. What is the primary mechanism by which stem cells from an umbilical cord transplant can survive in a mismatched recipient?

A. Higher tolerance to HLA mismatches
B. Increased dose of stem cells
C. Enhanced immune reconstitution
D. Lower risk of graft-versus-host disease (GVHD)

Q117. Which of the following cytokines is most crucial in the development of graft-versus-host disease (GVHD) after allogeneic stem cell transplantation?

A. Interferon-gamma (IFN-γ)
B. Interleukin-2 (IL-2)
C. Tumor necrosis factor-alpha (TNF-α)
D. Granulocyte-colony stimulating factor (G-CSF)

Q118. Which of the following strategies is most likely to prevent graft-versus-host disease (GVHD) after an allogeneic stem cell transplant?
A. Using autologous stem cells
B. Using a non-myeloablative conditioning regimen
C. Using immunosuppressive therapy to deplete T-cells
D. Using umbilical cord blood

Q119. Which of the following factors most directly influences the speed of immune reconstitution following an allogeneic stem cell transplant?
A. Donor age
B. Conditioning regimen intensity
C. Graft-versus-host disease (GVHD)
D. HLA matching

Q120. Which of the following is the most important consideration when selecting a donor for an allogeneic transplant?
A. The donor's age
B. The donor's gender
C. The degree of HLA matching
D. The donor's blood type

Q121. Which of the following is the most common source of stem cells for autologous transplantation?
A. Bone marrow
B. Peripheral blood
C. Umbilical cord blood
D. Placental blood

Q122. What is the primary purpose of using immunosuppressive therapy in allogeneic stem cell transplantation?
A. To promote graft-versus-tumor effect
B. To prevent graft-versus-host disease (GVHD)
C. To stimulate immune reconstitution
D. To eliminate residual malignant cells

Q123. Which of the following is a typical side effect of total body irradiation (TBI) used in the conditioning regimen for allogeneic stem cell transplantation?
A. Hair loss
B. Sepsis
C. Severe mucositis
D. Chronic kidney disease

Q124. Which of the following is a characteristic of autologous stem cell transplantation?
A. The patient receives stem cells from a matched donor
B. The patient's own stem cells are used
C. GVHD is a major complication
D. The patient must be immunosuppressed for life

Q125. Which of the following best describes the concept of "graft-versus-tumor (GvT) effect" in allogeneic stem cell transplantation?
A. Donor immune cells attack the recipient's healthy tissue

B. Donor immune cells attack the recipient's malignant cells
C. The recipient's immune system attacks the graft
D. The graft provides immune support for the recipient

Q126. Which of the following is the most common cause of infection in the early post-transplant period?
A. Bacterial infections
B. Fungal infections
C. Viral infections
D. Graft-versus-host disease

Q127. Which of the following statements best explains why graft-versus-host disease (GVHD) is more common in mismatched allogeneic stem cell transplants?
A. Donor immune cells recognize the recipient's tissues as foreign
B. The recipient's immune system attacks the graft
C. Donor immune cells suppress the recipient's immune response
D. The graft cannot survive in the recipient's body

Q128. Which of the following is the most significant factor in the speed of stem cell engraftment after an allogeneic stem cell transplant?
A. Donor age
B. Conditioning regimen intensity
C. Type of stem cell source used
D. HLA match between donor and recipient

Q129. Which of the following therapies is most commonly used to prevent graft-versus-host disease (GVHD) after an allogeneic stem cell transplant?
A. Antithymocyte globulin (ATG)
B. Rituximab
C. Methotrexate
D. Cyclophosphamide

Q130. Which of the following is a major advantage of using autologous stem cell transplantation for hematologic malignancies?
A. Reduced risk of graft-versus-host disease (GVHD)
B. Higher engraftment rates
C. No need for immunosuppressive therapy
D. Reduced risk of relapse

Q131. Which of the following cytokines is most important for the expansion and survival of T-cells in the graft-versus-tumor effect?
A. Interleukin-6 (IL-6)
B. Interleukin-2 (IL-2)
C. Tumor necrosis factor-alpha (TNF-α)
D. Granulocyte-colony stimulating factor (G-CSF)

Q132. Which stem cell source is most commonly used in pediatric allogeneic transplantation?
A. Bone marrow
B. Peripheral blood
C. Umbilical cord blood
D. Autologous stem cells

Q133. Which of the following is most likely to delay stem cell engraftment following an allogeneic stem cell transplant?
A. Fully matched donor
B. The use of G-CSF

C. Graft-versus-host disease (GVHD)
D. The use of autologous stem cells

Q134. Which of the following best explains the role of T-cells in the development of graft-versus-host disease (GVHD)?
A. T-cells from the recipient attack the donor's tissues
B. T-cells from the donor attack the recipient's tissues
C. T-cells from the recipient suppress the donor's immune response
D. T-cells from the donor attack the tumor cells in the recipient

Q135. Which of the following factors most significantly contributes to the risk of graft-versus-host disease (GVHD) in mismatched allogeneic stem cell transplants?
A. Donor age
B. Use of myeloablative conditioning
C. Degree of HLA mismatch
D. Type of stem cell source used

Q136. Which of the following best explains why the use of haploidentical stem cell transplantation is associated with a higher risk of graft-versus-host disease (GVHD)?
A. Incomplete HLA match between donor and recipient
B. The presence of high numbers of regulatory T-cells in the graft
C. The recipient's immune system is highly activated
D. The stem cells are from an unrelated donor

Q137. Which of the following factors is most important when selecting a stem cell source for pediatric allogeneic transplantation?
A. The donor's age
B. The degree of HLA match between donor and recipient
C. The recipient's weight
D. The recipient's previous exposure to chemotherapy

Q138. Which of the following interventions is commonly used to reduce the risk of graft failure after an allogeneic stem cell transplant?
A. T-cell depletion from the graft
B. Administration of high-dose chemotherapy
C. Increased dose of G-CSF
D. Use of cyclosporine for GVHD prevention

Q139. Which of the following is most likely to delay immune reconstitution after an allogeneic stem cell transplant?
A. Early administration of G-CSF
B. The development of graft-versus-host disease (GVHD)
C. The use of peripheral blood stem cells
D. Full HLA matching between donor and recipient

Q140. Which of the following is a major complication of using umbilical cord blood for allogeneic stem cell transplantation?
A. Increased risk of graft-versus-host disease (GVHD)
B. Delayed immune reconstitution
C. Higher risk of infection due to poor HLA matching
D. Faster engraftment compared to peripheral blood

Q141. Which of the following stem cell sources has the highest risk of graft rejection due to immunologic incompatibility?
A. Autologous stem cells
B. Matched sibling donor bone marrow

C. Umbilical cord blood
D. Unrelated donor peripheral blood stem cells

Q142. Which of the following best describes the function of granulocyte-colony stimulating factor (G-CSF) in stem cell mobilization?

A. To increase the production of neutrophils
B. To increase the production of platelets
C. To enhance the immune response
D. To reduce the risk of graft-versus-host disease

Q143. Which of the following is the most important factor in determining whether a patient is eligible for an allogeneic stem cell transplant?

A. Age of the patient
B. Type of hematologic disease
C. Availability of a matching donor
D. The patient's physical fitness for surgery

Q144. Which of the following complications is most commonly associated with high-dose chemotherapy in the conditioning regimen?

A. Severe mucositis
B. Graft-versus-host disease (GVHD)
C. Infection
D. Bone marrow suppression

Q145. What is the primary reason why graft-versus-tumor (GvT) effect is beneficial in allogeneic stem cell transplantation?

A. Donor T-cells attack the recipient's malignant cells
B. Donor T-cells suppress the recipient's immune system
C. Recipient immune cells attack the donor's cells
D. The graft acts as a source of immune recovery

Q146. Which of the following best describes the goal of using a myeloablative conditioning regimen in allogeneic stem cell transplantation?

A. To enhance the immune system of the recipient
B. To eliminate recipient hematopoietic cells and make room for donor cells
C. To reduce the risk of graft-versus-host disease
D. To stimulate the production of stem cells in the recipient

Q147. Which of the following is most likely to occur after using anti-thymocyte globulin (ATG) in an allogeneic stem cell transplant?

A. Increased risk of graft-versus-host disease (GVHD)
B. Increased immune reconstitution
C. Depletion of T-cells to reduce rejection and GVHD
D. Increased risk of infection due to immunosuppression

Q148. Which of the following factors is most likely to delay immune reconstitution after allogeneic stem cell transplantation?

A. Use of autologous stem cells
B. Fully matched donor
C. Development of graft-versus-host disease (GVHD)
D. High-dose chemotherapy in the conditioning regimen

Q149. Which of the following best describes the role of graft-versus-host disease (GVHD) in the outcome of an allogeneic stem cell transplant?

A. GVHD can help eliminate residual cancer cells by mediating the graft-versus-tumor effect
B. GVHD is a necessary part of the transplant process to promote immune reconstitution

C. GVHD is a complication that increases the risk of graft failure and infection
D. GVHD is a complication that only affects the skin and liver

Q150. What is the main difference between an autologous and an allogeneic stem cell transplant?
A. Autologous transplants use stem cells from a matched donor, while allogeneic transplants use the patient's own cells
B. Autologous transplants have a higher risk of graft-versus-host disease
C. Autologous transplants use the patient's own stem cells, while allogeneic transplants use stem cells from a donor
D. Allogeneic transplants require more immunosuppressive therapy than autologous transplants

Q151. Which of the following is the most common cause of graft failure in allogeneic stem cell transplantation?
A. Infection
B. Poor HLA matching
C. Graft-versus-host disease (GVHD)
D. Delayed immune reconstitution

Q152. Which of the following cytokines plays a key role in preventing graft rejection and promoting donor cell engraftment?
A. Interleukin-2 (IL-2)
B. Tumor necrosis factor-alpha (TNF-α)
C. Granulocyte-colony stimulating factor (G-CSF)
D. Interferon-gamma (IFN-γ)

Q153. What is the primary role of peripheral blood stem cell (PBSC) collection for autologous stem cell transplantation?
A. To treat graft-versus-host disease (GVHD)
B. To obtain a large number of stem cells for reinfusion
C. To enhance the immune response in the recipient
D. To prevent graft rejection by matching HLA

Q154. Which of the following is the main reason for using immunosuppressive drugs during the early post-transplant period?
A. To prevent graft-versus-host disease (GVHD)
B. To stimulate immune reconstitution
C. To reduce the risk of infection
D. To enhance graft-versus-tumor (GvT) effect

Q155. Which of the following is the primary challenge when using umbilical cord blood for allogeneic stem cell transplantation in adults?
A. Higher risk of graft-versus-host disease (GVHD)
B. Limited stem cell dose for adequate engraftment
C. Difficulty in HLA matching
D. Increased risk of graft rejection due to mismatched antigens

Q156. What is the main reason why peripheral blood stem cell (PBSC) transplantation is preferred over bone marrow transplantation in adults?
A. Higher rate of graft-versus-host disease (GVHD)
B. Faster stem cell engraftment
C. Lower HLA matching requirement
D. Lower infection risk

Q157. Which of the following is a key factor influencing the risk of graft-versus-host disease (GVHD) in unrelated donor allogeneic transplants?
A. Degree of HLA matching between donor and recipient

B. Age of the recipient
C. Donor's gender
D. Type of conditioning regimen used

Q158. Which of the following cytokines is most responsible for the graft-versus-tumor (GvT) effect in allogeneic stem cell transplantation?
A. Interleukin-10 (IL-10)
B. Interferon-gamma (IFN-γ)
C. Tumor necrosis factor-alpha (TNF-α)
D. Granulocyte-colony stimulating factor (G-CSF)

Q159. Which of the following is a major limitation of using umbilical cord blood for allogeneic stem cell transplantation in adults?
A. High risk of graft rejection
B. Low stem cell dose compared to peripheral blood
C. Difficulty in donor selection
D. Increased risk of infection due to immaturity of T-cells

Q160. Which of the following is most commonly used as a treatment for acute graft-versus-host disease (GVHD) in allogeneic stem cell transplant recipients?
A. Methotrexate
B. Cyclophosphamide
C. Steroids (e.g., prednisone)
D. Granulocyte-colony stimulating factor (G-CSF)

Q161. Which of the following is the most significant factor that influences the long-term success of hematopoietic stem cell transplantation?
A. The age of the donor
B. The quality of the conditioning regimen
C. The HLA match between donor and recipient
D. The patient's physical activity level

Q162. Which of the following is the primary risk associated with the use of high-dose chemotherapy in the conditioning regimen for hematopoietic stem cell transplantation?
A. Graft-versus-host disease (GVHD)
B. Severe mucositis and gastrointestinal toxicity
C. Increased risk of infection
D. Graft rejection due to inadequate stem cell dose

Q163. A 52-year-old patient undergoing autologous HSCT develops rigors and hypotension 10 minutes after infusion begins. The product was cryopreserved with DMSO. What should the nurse do first?
A. Stop the infusion and notify the physician
B. Administer corticosteroids immediately
C. Flush the line with saline and continue infusion
D. Check blood glucose level

Q164. A nurse notes that a patient's autologous stem cell product appears cloudy with clumps during thawing. What is the most appropriate nursing action?
A. Warm gently and continue infusion
B. Discard the product immediately
C. Return the product to the cell processing lab for evaluation
D. Filter the product through a standard blood filter

Q165. Following myeloablative conditioning, a 44-year-old patient reports severe mucositis and diarrhea. What is the nurse's priority intervention?
A. Encourage solid food intake

B. Provide opioid analgesia and maintain fluid balance
C. Hold all antibiotics until oral intake improves
D. Administer antidiarrheal agents immediately

Q166. A patient undergoing allogeneic transplantation receives total body irradiation (TBI). Which safety measure is most critical during nursing care?

A. Maintaining room humidity at 60%
B. Limiting staff exposure time and using shielding
C. Monitoring daily urine output
D. Avoiding metal jewelry

Q167. During stem cell collection, apheresis flow alarms repeatedly occur. What initial action should the nurse take?

A. Adjust the anticoagulant ratio
B. Reposition the venous access and check line patency
C. Stop the collection immediately
D. Flush the system with saline

Q168. A patient complains of a garlic-like odor and taste during stem cell infusion. What should the nurse explain?

A. This indicates bacterial contamination
B. It results from DMSO used as a cryoprotectant
C. It reflects electrolyte imbalance
D. It signifies infusion reaction requiring cessation

Q169. A stem cell infusion is delayed by four hours due to equipment malfunction. The cells remain at room temperature. What should the nurse do?

A. Proceed with infusion
B. Re-freeze the cells for later use
C. Contact the cell processing lab for product viability testing
D. Place the bag in ice water until infusion resumes

Q170. A patient develops facial flushing and dyspnea halfway through an allogeneic cell infusion. Which immediate medication is typically indicated?

A. Acetaminophen
B. Hydrocortisone or antihistamine
C. Morphine sulfate
D. Calcium gluconate

Q171. Which patient factor most influences selection of a reduced-intensity conditioning (RIC) regimen?

A. High performance status
B. Older age or comorbidities limiting tolerance
C. Early-stage disease
D. HLA-matched sibling donor availability

Q172. Apheresis monitoring reveals hypocalcemia symptoms during collection. What should the nurse anticipate?

A. Infusion of calcium gluconate
B. Stopping anticoagulant administration
C. Increasing citrate flow rate
D. Starting a vasopressor

Q173. Which intervention minimizes risk of bacterial contamination during marrow harvest?

A. Using sterile technique and laminar airflow environment
B. Adding antibiotics to marrow product

C. Shortening collection time to less than one hour
D. Storing product at room temperature overnight

Q174. A nurse notes that a patient's urine turns pinkish during stem cell infusion. Which explanation is correct?

A. Hemolysis from DMSO and rapid thawing
B. Early hemorrhagic cystitis
C. Renal failure onset
D. Contamination from donor cells

Q175. A patient reports chest tightness and coughing during cellular infusion. Oxygen saturation drops to 89%. What is the nurse's next action?

A. Continue infusion at slower rate
B. Stop infusion and administer oxygen
C. Give intravenous fluids rapidly
D. Notify lab to recheck product viability

Q176. Which of the following conditioning agents primarily causes hepatic veno-occlusive disease (VOD)?

A. Melphalan
B. Busulfan
C. Cyclophosphamide
D. Etoposide

Q177. A nurse educates a donor about granulocyte colony-stimulating factor (G-CSF). What key teaching point should be emphasized?

A. It reduces infection risk permanently
B. It mobilizes stem cells into peripheral blood for collection
C. It prevents graft-versus-host disease
D. It suppresses immune response

Q178. Which sign during infusion indicates DMSO toxicity rather than mild reaction?

A. Nausea
B. Hypertension and bradycardia
C. Transient flushing
D. Garlic odor

Q179. A patient receiving a mismatched unrelated donor graft develops back pain during infusion. What is the nurse's first priority?

A. Assess for hemolytic transfusion reaction
B. Increase infusion rate
C. Give analgesics and continue
D. Check vital signs every hour

Q180. When preparing to infuse fresh, non-cryopreserved stem cells, what key nursing verification is required?

A. Crossmatch result and product labeling
B. Presence of DMSO
C. Thawing temperature accuracy
D. Date of last chemotherapy

Q181. A patient receiving a CAR-T cell infusion experiences fever, hypotension, and tachycardia 6 hours post-infusion. What is the most likely cause?

A. Bacterial sepsis
B. Cytokine release syndrome (CRS)
C. Allergic infusion reaction

D. DMSO intolerance

Q182. During preparative chemotherapy, a patient's absolute neutrophil count drops below 500/µL. Which nursing intervention takes priority?

A. Encourage fresh fruit intake

B. Maintain protective isolation and strict hand hygiene

C. Begin physical therapy

D. Delay all conditioning drugs

Q183. During autologous transplantation, the patient develops tingling of lips and fingers during apheresis. Which nursing action is most appropriate?

A. Stop collection immediately

B. Administer calcium gluconate intravenously

C. Increase citrate infusion rate

D. Apply warm blankets

Q184. A 60-year-old undergoing reduced-intensity conditioning develops confusion and ataxia after busulfan. What nursing action is most urgent?

A. Document and continue observation

B. Notify provider for possible seizure prophylaxis adjustment

C. Give IV fluids immediately

D. Reduce room lighting and provide rest

Q185. A nurse prepares to infuse cryopreserved stem cells. Which pre-medication combination best minimizes reactions?

A. Acetaminophen, diphenhydramine, and corticosteroid

B. Morphine and lorazepam

C. Ondansetron only

D. Heparin flush and antibiotic prophylaxis

Q186. During thawing, a nurse notices rapid warming above 40 °C. What is the appropriate next step?

A. Discard and notify processing lab

B. Continue thawing until complete

C. Cool rapidly in ice water

D. Proceed with infusion immediately

Q187. A patient reports shortness of breath and back pain minutes after allogeneic infusion begins. Which is the nurse's first action?

A. Increase oxygen and slow infusion

B. Stop infusion and maintain IV access with saline

C. Administer furosemide

D. Send product for sterility testing

Q188. Which nursing measure reduces patient risk for line-related infection during stem-cell collection?

A. Changing central-line dressings with sterile technique

B. Using prophylactic antibiotics daily

C. Keeping line open with heparinized saline continuously

D. Flushing only at start and end of collection

Q189. After melphalan conditioning, a patient experiences oral ulcerations with difficulty eating. What is the most appropriate nursing intervention?

A. Offer carbonated beverages for relief

B. Implement saline/bicarbonate mouth rinses and topical analgesia

C. Encourage hard foods to desensitize mucosa

D. Reduce fluid intake to minimize pain

Q190. A stem-cell product arrives labeled for another patient with a similar name. What should the nurse do?
A. Proceed if date of birth matches
B. Verify with lab and hold infusion
C. Relabel the bag correctly
D. Ask another nurse to double-check and proceed
Q191. A patient undergoing donor lymphocyte infusion develops fever and rash within 24 hours. Which complication should the nurse suspect?
A. Cytokine release syndrome
B. Acute GVHD onset
C. Infectious febrile episode
D. Engraftment syndrome
Q192. A donor develops splenic pain after several days of G-CSF. What is the most appropriate nursing instruction?
A. Apply warm compresses
B. Seek immediate medical evaluation for possible splenic rupture
C. Continue G-CSF and monitor pain
D. Use over-the-counter analgesics only
Q193. A patient undergoing allogeneic transplant develops hematuria during cyclophosphamide therapy. Which preventive measure should have been emphasized?
A. Forced diuresis with mesna
B. Antifungal prophylaxis
C. Antihypertensive therapy
D. Cranberry juice intake
Q194. During product infusion, the nurse detects chest tightness and wheezing. Which medication should be prepared first?
A. Epinephrine
B. Diphenhydramine
C. Methylprednisolone
D. Furosemide
Q195. The nurse notes a sharp rise in the patient's temperature during infusion of thawed cells. What is the best immediate action?
A. Stop infusion and evaluate for reaction
B. Give acetaminophen and continue
C. Check vital signs after completion
D. Increase infusion speed
Q196. Apheresis yields show low CD34+ count after first collection. What should the nurse anticipate?
A. Proceed with transplantation
B. Notify physician for additional G-CSF or collection day
C. Store product and infuse anyway
D. Add donor plasma to increase concentration
Q197. A patient receiving total body irradiation expresses anxiety about sterility precautions. What should the nurse emphasize?
A. TBI requires isolation to protect staff
B. Protective isolation prevents infection while immune system is ablated
C. Lead-shielding rooms eliminate all radiation risk
D. Visitors may enter freely once treatment begins

Q198. During infusion, the patient experiences nausea, bradycardia, and elevated blood pressure. What complication is most likely?

A. DMSO toxicity

B. Bacterial contamination

C. Transfusion-related sepsis

D. Delayed hemolysis

Q199. Which action prevents cryopreserved cell bag rupture during thawing?

A. Immerse sealed bag in 37 °C water bath with continuous agitation

B. Thaw at room temperature for 20 minutes

C. Open bag to release gas before thawing

D. Shake vigorously after immersion

Q200. A patient's vital signs show hypertension during infusion of cryopreserved cells. What is the nurse's priority?

A. Continue infusion and recheck after 15 min

B. Slow rate and assess for DMSO-related reaction

C. Stop infusion and discard product

D. Administer diuretics

Answer key and Explanation (101-200)

Q101. Answer: B

Explanation: Umbilical cord blood has fewer T cells, which significantly reduces the risk of GVHD. Option A – cord blood typically contains fewer stem cells than peripheral blood. Option C – engraftment is typically slower with cord blood. Option D – cord blood has a more relaxed HLA match requirement.
SubChapter: D. Sources of stem cells — Umbilical cord blood

Q102. Answer: C

Explanation: HLA compatibility plays a critical role in the development of GVHD, with mismatched grafts increasing risk. Option A – infection risk is influenced by immunosuppression and recovery, not HLA alone. Option B – graft rejection is minimized by better HLA matching but not fully determined by it. Option D – engraftment speed is affected by multiple factors, not just HLA.
SubChapter: H. Donor selection, care, and education

Q103. Answer: B

Explanation: Serologic testing for EBV, CMV, and other latent viruses is crucial in assessing infection risks in transplant candidates. Option A – bone marrow biopsy is used for disease staging, not infection screening. Option C – pulmonary function tests assess lung capacity, not infection risk. Option D – echocardiogram assesses heart function, not infection.
SubChapter: E. Recipient suitability and evaluation

Q104. Answer: D

Explanation: TBI is used to eliminate the recipient's hematopoietic cells to make space for donor cell engraftment. Option A – GVHD is managed with immunosuppressants, not TBI. Option B – TBI also suppresses the immune system, but its primary role is cell elimination. Option C – TBI itself does not directly enhance engraftment.
SubChapter: C. Conditioning / preparative regimens

Q105. Answer: B

Explanation: Haploidentical transplants carry a higher risk of GVHD due to incomplete HLA matching. Option A – stem cell availability is not the main challenge in haploidentical transplants. Option C – HLA matching is a challenge but not the primary factor affecting outcomes. Option D – immune reconstitution is slower but not the primary problem.
SubChapter: C. Types of transplants — Haploidentical

Q106. Answer: C

Explanation: T lymphocytes from the donor attack the recipient's tissues, initiating GVHD. Option A – B lymphocytes are involved in antibody production, not GVHD. Option B – neutrophils are essential in early infection responses, not GVHD. Option D – monocytes help with inflammation but don't initiate GVHD.
SubChapter: A. Immune system and function

Q107. Answer: C

Explanation: Bone pain is a common side effect of G-CSF, a mobilization agent used to increase stem cell numbers. Option A – graft rejection is not a concern in autologous transplantation. Option B – neutropenia occurs during conditioning, not mobilization. Option D – liver toxicity is not commonly associated with stem cell mobilization.
SubChapter: D. Stem cell mobilization

Q108. Answer: A

Explanation: Autologous stem cells eliminate the risk of GVHD since the patient's own cells are used. Option B – engraftment rates are similar in autologous and allogeneic transplants. Option C – infection

risk is still significant post-transplant. Option D – immune tolerance is a concern in allogeneic grafts, not autologous.
SubChapter: C. Types of transplants — Autologous

Q109. Answer: B

Explanation: Infection due to immunosuppression is the leading cause of early graft failure in allogeneic transplants. Option A – GVHD affects graft function later. Option C – poor HLA matching primarily increases the risk of rejection, not early graft failure. Option D – delayed immune reconstitution occurs over time, not in the early phase.
SubChapter: A. Cellular goals of therapy

Q110. Answer: A

Explanation: Cyclophosphamide depletes host immune cells to reduce the risk of graft rejection. Option B – cyclophosphamide does not activate donor immune cells in this context. Option C – it does not directly enhance engraftment. Option D – cyclophosphamide suppresses the host immune system, including T-cells, to prevent rejection.
SubChapter: C. Conditioning / preparative regimens

Q111. Answer: C

Explanation: T-cells mediate the graft-versus-tumor (GvT) effect by recognizing and attacking residual tumor cells. Option A – T-cells can contribute to GVHD, but their main role is the GvT effect. Option B – T-cells are not primarily involved in infection prevention. Option D – T-cells help with immune reconstitution, but GvT is their primary function.
SubChapter: A. Immune system and function

Q112. Answer: B

Explanation: Infection is the leading cause of death in the early post-transplant period due to immunosuppression. Option A – graft rejection is less common in well-matched grafts. Option C – GVHD develops later and can be managed with immunosuppressants. Option D – relapse occurs later in the post-transplant phase.
SubChapter: III. Infection prevention and management

Q113. Answer: B

Explanation: ATG depletes recipient T-cells to reduce the risk of graft rejection. Option A – ATG is not used to stimulate immune reconstitution. Option C – ATG reduces T-cell activity, which could suppress GvT. Option D – ATG does not directly reduce infection risk.
SubChapter: H. Donor selection, care and education

Q114. Answer: A

Explanation: Bone pain is a common complication of PBSC collection due to G-CSF stimulation. Option B – anemia is not commonly associated with PBSC collection. Option C – platelet deficiency is not a typical complication. Option D – GVHD occurs after transplant, not during PBSC collection.
SubChapter: D. Stem cell mobilization

Q115. Answer: D

Explanation: Unrelated donor peripheral blood stem cells have a higher risk of graft rejection due to HLA mismatch. Option A – autologous stem cells cannot be rejected. Option B – bone marrow from a matched sibling is well-matched and has a lower risk of rejection. Option C – umbilical cord blood has a lower risk of rejection due to its immunologic characteristics.
SubChapter: C. Types of transplants

Q116. Answer: A

Explanation: Umbilical cord blood has higher tolerance to HLA mismatches due to the immaturity of its immune cells. Option B – cord blood typically has a lower stem cell dose. Option C – immune reconstitution is slower with cord blood. Option D – while cord blood has lower GVHD risk, its primary advantage is HLA mismatch tolerance.

SubChapter: D. Sources of stem cells

Q117. Answer: A

Explanation: IFN-γ plays a critical role in the pathogenesis of GVHD by activating cytotoxic T-cells. Option B – IL-2 promotes T-cell proliferation, but IFN-γ is more critical for GVHD. Option C – TNF-α contributes to inflammation, but IFN-γ is a more potent driver of GVHD. Option D – G-CSF is used for stem cell mobilization, not for GVHD.

SubChapter: A. Immune system and function

Q118. Answer: C

Explanation: Immunosuppressive therapy, including T-cell depletion, is the most effective strategy for preventing GVHD. Option A – autologous stem cells cannot cause GVHD. Option B – non-myeloablative regimens are not typically used to prevent GVHD. Option D – umbilical cord blood does lower the risk of GVHD, but T-cell depletion is more effective.

SubChapter: C. Conditioning / preparative regimens

Q119. Answer: C

Explanation: GVHD significantly delays immune reconstitution by damaging the recipient's immune system. Option A – donor age affects outcomes but not the speed of immune reconstitution. Option B – while conditioning regimen intensity affects engraftment, GVHD has a more direct impact on immune recovery. Option D – HLA matching affects graft rejection, not immune reconstitution speed.

SubChapter: A. Cellular goals of therapy

Q120. Answer: C

Explanation: HLA matching is the most important factor in reducing the risk of graft rejection and GVHD. Option A – donor age can affect outcomes, but HLA compatibility is the primary consideration. Option B – gender affects graft rejection but is secondary to HLA matching. Option D – blood type compatibility is less important than HLA matching.

SubChapter: H. Donor selection, care and education

Q121. Answer: B

Explanation: Peripheral blood stem cells are most commonly used for autologous transplantation because they provide faster engraftment. Option A – bone marrow is also used, but less commonly in autologous transplants. Option C – cord blood is not typically used in adults for autologous transplantation. Option D – placental blood is not a standard source.

SubChapter: D. Sources of stem cells

Q122. Answer: B

Explanation: Immunosuppressive therapy is primarily used to prevent graft-versus-host disease (GVHD) after allogeneic stem cell transplantation. Option A – GvT effect is mediated by donor immune cells, not immunosuppressive therapy. Option C – immune reconstitution occurs naturally after transplant. Option D – residual tumor cells are eliminated through other therapies.

SubChapter: A. Immune system and function

Q123. Answer: C

Explanation: Severe mucositis is a common side effect of TBI due to damage to the gastrointestinal mucosa. Option A – hair loss can occur but is not the primary side effect of TBI. Option B – sepsis can occur but is more commonly associated with neutropenia. Option D – chronic kidney disease is not a common immediate side effect of TBI.

SubChapter: C. Conditioning / preparative regimens

Q124. Answer: B

Explanation: Autologous stem cell transplantation involves using the patient's own stem cells, eliminating the risk of graft-versus-host disease (GVHD). Option A – allogeneic transplants use stem cells from a donor. Option C – GVHD is not a concern with autologous transplantation. Option D – immunosuppression is temporary in autologous transplants, unlike in allogeneic transplants.

SubChapter: C. Types of transplants — Autologous

Q125. Answer: B

Explanation: GvT effect occurs when donor immune cells recognize and attack residual tumor cells in the recipient. Option A – donor immune cells attack the recipient's healthy tissue in GVHD, not GvT. Option C – the recipient's immune system attacks the graft in rejection, not GvT. Option D – the graft provides immune cells but is not the main immune support in GvT.

SubChapter: A. Cellular goals of therapy

Q126. Answer: A

Explanation: Bacterial infections are the most common due to neutropenia from chemotherapy and conditioning regimens. Option B – fungal infections are common but less frequent than bacterial infections. Option C – viral infections are a concern but typically occur later. Option D – GVHD is an immune complication, not an infection.

SubChapter: III. Infection prevention and management

Q127. Answer: A

Explanation: In mismatched transplants, donor immune cells recognize the recipient's tissues as foreign and attack them, leading to GVHD. Option B – the recipient's immune system attacking the graft occurs in graft rejection, not GVHD. Option C – donor immune cells suppress the recipient's immune response to prevent GVHD. Option D – mismatched grafts are more likely to fail, but GVHD is caused by immune attack.

SubChapter: A. Immune system and function

Q128. Answer: D

Explanation: HLA matching is the most significant factor in the speed of engraftment, with better matches leading to faster engraftment. Option A – donor age can influence outcomes but is secondary to HLA matching. Option B – conditioning regimen intensity affects engraftment but is not the primary factor. Option C – the type of stem cell source influences engraftment but not as much as HLA matching.

SubChapter: A. Cellular goals of therapy

Q129. Answer: C

Explanation: Methotrexate is commonly used in combination with other drugs to prevent GVHD after allogeneic transplantation. Option A – ATG is used to deplete T-cells, not directly prevent GVHD. Option B – rituximab targets B cells, not T cells involved in GVHD. Option D – cyclophosphamide is used in conditioning, not GVHD prevention.

SubChapter: A. Cellular goals of therapy

Q130. Answer: A

Explanation: The main advantage of autologous stem cell transplantation is the elimination of GVHD, as the patient's own cells are used. Option B – autologous transplants typically have similar engraftment rates to allogeneic transplants. Option C – immunosuppressive therapy is still required post-transplant to prevent complications. Option D – relapse rates may still occur depending on the disease type.

SubChapter: C. Types of transplants — Autologous

Q131. Answer: B

Explanation: Interleukin-2 (IL-2) is critical for the proliferation and survival of T-cells, which mediate the graft-versus-tumor (GvT) effect. Option A – IL-6 is involved in inflammation, but IL-2 is key for T-cell survival. Option C – TNF-α promotes inflammation but is less involved in GvT. Option D – G-CSF is used for stem cell mobilization, not GvT.

SubChapter: A. Immune system and function

Q132. Answer: C

Explanation: Umbilical cord blood is commonly used in pediatric transplants due to its better immunologic characteristics and ease of collection. Option A – bone marrow is less frequently used in

children. Option B – peripheral blood is more common in adults. Option D – autologous stem cells are not used in allogeneic transplantation.
SubChapter: D. Sources of stem cells

Q133. Answer: C

Explanation: GVHD can delay stem cell engraftment by causing immune-mediated damage to the graft. Option A – fully matched donors typically lead to faster engraftment. Option B – G-CSF is used to promote faster engraftment. Option D – autologous stem cells are not associated with engraftment delay.
SubChapter: A. Cellular goals of therapy

Q134. Answer: B

Explanation: GVHD occurs when T-cells from the donor attack the recipient's tissues, recognizing them as foreign. Option A – GVHD is mediated by donor T-cells, not the recipient's. Option C – T-cells from the recipient are involved in immune rejection, not suppression. Option D – donor T-cells mediate the graft-versus-tumor (GvT) effect, not GVHD.
SubChapter: A. Immune system and function

Q135. Answer: C

Explanation: The degree of HLA mismatch between donor and recipient is the most significant factor in the development of GVHD. Option A – donor age affects other outcomes but not GVHD risk directly. Option B – myeloablative conditioning reduces GVHD risk by eliminating the recipient's immune system. Option D – stem cell source impacts engraftment but not directly GVHD.
SubChapter: H. Donor selection, care, and education

Q136. Answer: A

Explanation: Haploidentical transplants involve a partial HLA match, which increases the risk of GVHD due to immune incompatibility. Option B – regulatory T-cells typically reduce GVHD risk, not increase it. Option C – the recipient's immune activation is not the primary cause of GVHD in haploidentical transplants. Option D – unrelated donor transplants may carry risks, but haploidentical transplants have higher GVHD risk due to HLA mismatch.
SubChapter: C. Types of transplants — Haploidentical

Q137. Answer: B

Explanation: The degree of HLA matching is the most important factor in stem cell selection for pediatric transplants to reduce the risk of rejection and GVHD. Option A – donor age influences outcomes but is not as crucial as HLA match. Option C – recipient weight is not the primary factor in stem cell source selection. Option D – prior chemotherapy affects conditioning regimens, not stem cell source selection.
SubChapter: H. Donor selection, care, and education

Q138. Answer: A

Explanation: T-cell depletion from the graft reduces the risk of graft failure by decreasing the chances of host-versus-graft reactions. Option B – high-dose chemotherapy is used for conditioning but not to prevent graft failure. Option C – G-CSF is used to mobilize stem cells, not to prevent graft failure. Option D – cyclosporine is used for GVHD prevention but doesn't directly prevent graft failure.
SubChapter: A. Cellular goals of therapy

Q139. Answer: B

Explanation: GVHD delays immune reconstitution by damaging both the donor's and recipient's immune systems. Option A – G-CSF accelerates stem cell mobilization and engraftment but does not delay immune reconstitution. Option C – peripheral blood stem cells can lead to faster engraftment. Option D – full HLA matching typically promotes faster immune recovery.
SubChapter: A. Cellular goals of therapy

Q140. Answer: B

Explanation: Umbilical cord blood has lower stem cell content, which leads to slower immune reconstitution. Option A – cord blood has a lower risk of GVHD due to fewer T-cells. Option C – cord blood has a more relaxed HLA matching requirement, reducing the risk of rejection. Option D – engraftment is typically slower with cord blood compared to peripheral blood.
SubChapter: D. Sources of stem cells — Umbilical cord blood

Q141. Answer: D

Explanation: Unrelated donor peripheral blood stem cells have the highest risk of graft rejection due to immunologic differences. Option A – autologous stem cells cannot be rejected. Option B – matched sibling bone marrow has the lowest risk of rejection. Option C – umbilical cord blood has a lower risk of rejection.
SubChapter: C. Types of transplants

Q142. Answer: A

Explanation: G-CSF is used to stimulate the production of neutrophils and mobilize stem cells into peripheral blood. Option B – platelets are produced by megakaryocytes, not G-CSF. Option C – G-CSF enhances neutrophil production, not the overall immune response. Option D – G-CSF does not prevent GVHD.
SubChapter: D. Stem cell mobilization

Q143. Answer: C

Explanation: The availability of a matching donor is critical for an allogeneic transplant. Option A – age can affect transplant eligibility but is not the most important factor. Option B – the type of disease affects transplant eligibility, but donor match is crucial. Option D – physical fitness is important but secondary to donor availability.
SubChapter: E. Recipient suitability and evaluation

Q144. Answer: D

Explanation: High-dose chemotherapy causes bone marrow suppression, which is why stem cell transplantation is necessary. Option A – mucositis occurs but is less common than bone marrow suppression. Option B – GVHD is a complication of allogeneic transplant but not directly from chemotherapy. Option C – infection is common, but bone marrow suppression is the direct result of high-dose chemotherapy.
SubChapter: C. Conditioning / preparative regimens

Q145. Answer: A

Explanation: The GvT effect occurs when donor T-cells attack and kill the recipient's tumor cells. Option B – donor T-cells may cause GVHD, but this suppresses the immune system, not the tumor. Option C – the recipient's immune cells are not involved in GvT. Option D – immune recovery is important but not the main goal of GvT.
SubChapter: A. Cellular goals of therapy

Q146. Answer: B

Explanation: Myeloablative conditioning eliminates the recipient's hematopoietic cells to allow for donor stem cell engraftment. Option A – immune suppression is not the primary goal of conditioning. Option C – GVHD is prevented by immunosuppressive therapy, not conditioning. Option D – conditioning does not stimulate stem cell production in the recipient.
SubChapter: C. Conditioning / preparative regimens

Q147. Answer: C

Explanation: ATG depletes T-cells to reduce the risk of graft rejection and GVHD. Option A – ATG is used to reduce GVHD, not increase it. Option B – ATG suppresses the immune response, slowing reconstitution. Option D – while ATG does suppress the immune system, its primary goal is T-cell depletion, not infection control.
SubChapter: H. Donor selection, care, and education

Q148. Answer: C
Explanation: GVHD delays immune reconstitution by causing immune damage to the recipient's tissues. Option A – autologous stem cells do not lead to immune delay as much as allogeneic transplants. Option B – full HLA matching promotes faster immune recovery. Option D – high-dose chemotherapy affects engraftment but not immune reconstitution as much as GVHD.
SubChapter: A. Cellular goals of therapy
Q149. Answer: C
Explanation: GVHD is an immune complication that can increase the risk of graft failure and infection due to required immunosuppression. Option A – GvT effect is beneficial, but GVHD is not the primary mechanism. Option B – GVHD is not a necessary process but an unwanted complication. Option D – GVHD can affect multiple organs, not just the skin and liver.
SubChapter: A. Immune system and function
Q150. Answer: C
Explanation: Autologous transplants use the patient's own stem cells, while allogeneic transplants use stem cells from a donor. Option A – this is the reverse of the actual transplant types. Option B – GVHD occurs only in allogeneic transplants. Option D – allogeneic transplants do require more immunosuppression, but that's secondary to the stem cell source difference.
SubChapter: C. Types of transplants
Q151. Answer: B
Explanation: Poor HLA matching is the most common cause of graft failure in allogeneic stem cell transplants due to immune rejection. Option A – infection contributes to complications but not directly to graft failure. Option C – GVHD can impair function but doesn't directly cause failure. Option D – immune reconstitution is delayed but typically does not cause immediate graft failure.
SubChapter: A. Cellular goals of therapy
Q152. Answer: A
Explanation: IL-2 is critical for promoting T-cell expansion and helping donor cells engraft in the recipient. Option B – TNF-α is involved in inflammation but not directly in engraftment. Option C – G-CSF is used to mobilize stem cells but doesn't directly affect engraftment. Option D – IFN-γ is involved in immune responses but not engraftment promotion.
SubChapter: A. Immune system and function
Q153. Answer: B
Explanation: PBSC collection is used to obtain a large number of stem cells for reinfusion during autologous transplantation. Option A – PBSC is not used to treat GVHD, which is more relevant to allogeneic transplants. Option C – PBSC doesn't enhance the recipient's immune response. Option D – HLA matching is primarily relevant to allogeneic transplants.
SubChapter: D. Stem cell mobilization
Q154. Answer: A
Explanation: Immunosuppressive drugs are used to prevent GVHD in the early post-transplant period. Option B – immunosuppressive therapy does not stimulate immune reconstitution. Option C – immunosuppressives increase infection risk, so antibiotics are used for infection prevention. Option D – GvT is mediated by donor immune cells, not by immunosuppressive therapy.
SubChapter: A. Cellular goals of therapy
Q155. Answer: B
Explanation: Umbilical cord blood has a lower stem cell dose, which can limit engraftment success in adults. Option A – cord blood has a lower risk of GVHD due to fewer T-cells. Option C – HLA matching requirements for cord blood are less stringent than other sources. Option D – mismatched antigens are less of a concern with cord blood than with other stem cell sources.
SubChapter: D. Sources of stem cells — Umbilical cord blood

Q156. Answer: B
Explanation: PBSC transplantation is preferred in adults due to faster stem cell engraftment. Option A – PBSC transplants are associated with higher GVHD risk, not lower. Option C – HLA matching requirements are similar for both PBSC and bone marrow. Option D – infection risk is influenced by other factors, not by stem cell source alone.
SubChapter: D. Sources of stem cells
Q157. Answer: A
Explanation: The degree of HLA matching between donor and recipient is the key factor influencing GVHD risk in unrelated donor transplants. Option B – recipient age affects outcomes but not the primary risk for GVHD. Option C – gender differences can contribute to GVHD risk, but HLA mismatch is more significant. Option D – conditioning regimen affects GVHD risk but is not the main factor.
SubChapter: H. Donor selection, care, and education
Q158. Answer: B
Explanation: Interferon-gamma (IFN-γ) is a key cytokine in activating donor T-cells to mediate the graft-versus-tumor (GvT) effect. Option A – IL-10 suppresses immune responses, which would not promote GvT. Option C – TNF-α is involved in inflammation but not directly in GvT. Option D – G-CSF is used to mobilize stem cells, not for GvT.
SubChapter: A. Immune system and function
Q159. Answer: B
Explanation: The main limitation of using umbilical cord blood in adults is the low stem cell dose, which may lead to slower engraftment. Option A – the risk of graft rejection is lower in cord blood than other sources. Option C – donor selection is easier due to relaxed HLA matching. Option D – T-cell immaturity in cord blood actually reduces the risk of GVHD, not infection.
SubChapter: D. Sources of stem cells — Umbilical cord blood
Q160. Answer: C
Explanation: Steroids (e.g., prednisone) are the most commonly used treatment for acute GVHD to reduce inflammation and immune response. Option A – methotrexate is used to prevent GVHD, not treat it. Option B – cyclophosphamide is used in conditioning regimens, not for treating GVHD. Option D – G-CSF is used for stem cell mobilization, not for treating GVHD.
SubChapter: A. Immune system and function
Q161. Answer: C
Explanation: The HLA match between donor and recipient is the most significant factor influencing the long-term success of the transplant. Option A – donor age affects outcomes but is less significant than HLA match. Option B – conditioning regimens are important but the quality of HLA matching is more critical. Option D – physical activity level can help recovery but does not significantly impact transplant success.
SubChapter: H. Donor selection, care and education
Q162. Answer: B
Explanation: High-dose chemotherapy is associated with severe mucositis and gastrointestinal toxicity due to its effect on rapidly dividing cells. Option A – GVHD is not caused by chemotherapy but by immune reaction post-transplant. Option C – infection risk is increased by immunosuppression but is not the primary risk of chemotherapy. Option D – stem cell dose is managed separately from chemotherapy.
SubChapter: C. Conditioning / preparative regimens
Q163. Answer: A
Explanation: Acute infusion reactions to cryoprotectant DMSO can trigger vasovagal and anaphylactoid responses. Immediate cessation prevents worsening of hypotension and airway compromise. Option B is supportive but follows stabilization. Option C risks further exposure. Option D is unrelated to infusion reaction management.

SubChapter: Cellular infusion management
Q164. Answer: C
Explanation: Clumping suggests cryopreservation damage or thawing error; returning the product ensures viability testing and prevents infusion of hemolyzed cells. Warming alone could worsen integrity. Discarding prematurely wastes viable product. Standard filters are inappropriate for stem cell infusions.
SubChapter: Product collection and storage integrity
Q165. Answer: B
Explanation: Mucositis and diarrhea after high-dose conditioning reflect cytotoxic mucosal injury. Analgesia maintains comfort, and hydration prevents renal toxicity from drug excretion. Antidiarrheals (D) risk ileus; withholding antibiotics (C) heightens infection risk; solid foods (A) exacerbate injury.
SubChapter: Conditioning regimen management
Q166. Answer: B
Explanation: Radiation safety is paramount during TBI to minimize staff and patient exposure; time, distance, and shielding principles apply. Other options are general comfort or hygiene measures but not directly linked to radiation protection standards.
SubChapter: Conditioning therapy – radiation safety
Q167. Answer: B
Explanation: Most apheresis flow issues stem from catheter malposition or kinking; repositioning restores flow safely. Stopping collection may be premature; anticoagulant adjustment affects yield only after mechanical causes are excluded. Saline flushing is secondary.
SubChapter: Stem cell product collection procedures
Q168. Answer: B
Explanation: Dimethyl sulfoxide (DMSO) causes transient odor and taste changes as it volatilizes through lungs. It is benign but unpleasant; reassurance is key. It does not signal contamination (A) or reaction (D); electrolyte imbalance (C) is unrelated.
SubChapter: Cryopreserved infusion effects
Q169. Answer: C
Explanation: Cell viability declines rapidly at room temperature; lab evaluation ensures hematopoietic potential before reinfusion. Cooling or refreezing without control can damage cells. Proceeding without confirmation risks engraftment failure.
SubChapter: Product handling and viability
Q170. Answer: B
Explanation: Allergic-type reactions from cryoprotectants or donor plasma respond to antihistamines or corticosteroids. Prompt administration reduces progression to anaphylaxis. Analgesics (C) or acetaminophen (A) are supportive only; calcium (D) addresses citrate toxicity, not hypersensitivity.
SubChapter: Infusion-related reactions
Q171. Answer: B
Explanation: RIC regimens minimize toxicity for older or fragile patients who cannot tolerate myeloablative doses while preserving graft-versus-tumor effects. High performance status favors standard intensity. Disease stage or donor match influence other aspects, not regimen intensity.
SubChapter: Conditioning regimen intensity selection
Q172. Answer: A
Explanation: Citrate anticoagulant binds calcium, causing perioral tingling and tetany; calcium supplementation corrects it quickly. Reducing anticoagulant (B) can clot the circuit; vasopressors (D) are unnecessary unless severe hypotension occurs.
SubChapter: Collection-related metabolic management
Q173. Answer: A

Explanation: Strict asepsis and laminar airflow reduce contamination risk. Adding antibiotics post-collection compromises cell viability; shortened time (C) may reduce yield; room-temperature storage fosters bacterial growth.
SubChapter: Harvest sterility protocols

Q174. Answer: A

Explanation: Mild hemoglobinuria occurs from red cell lysis during cryopreserved cell thawing; transient and self-limited. Monitoring and hydration suffice. Hemorrhagic cystitis (B) occurs later post-conditioning, not during infusion.
SubChapter: Infusion-related complications

Q175. Answer: B

Explanation: Acute pulmonary reactions require stopping infusion and oxygen support to prevent respiratory distress. Fluid bolus worsens pulmonary congestion; viability testing is irrelevant mid-infusion.
SubChapter: Acute infusion reactions

Q176. Answer: B

Explanation: Busulfan leads to endothelial injury and hepatic sinusoidal obstruction, hallmark of VOD. Monitoring bilirubin and weight gain detects early toxicity. Cyclophosphamide causes cystitis; melphalan mainly affects mucosa; etoposide induces myelosuppression.
SubChapter: Chemotherapy conditioning toxicity

Q177. Answer: B

Explanation: G-CSF promotes release of CD34+ stem cells from marrow to circulation, enabling efficient apheresis. It is transient and reversible. It neither prevents GVHD nor causes lasting immune suppression.
SubChapter: Mobilization and collection principles

Q178. Answer: B

Explanation: Severe DMSO toxicity manifests with cardiovascular instability (hypertension/bradycardia), requiring immediate cessation and monitoring. Other listed symptoms are common benign effects of DMSO.
SubChapter: Cryoprotectant toxicity management

Q179. Answer: A

Explanation: Back pain signals hemolysis from ABO incompatibility in mismatched infusions; urgent assessment prevents acute renal failure and shock. Continuing infusion risks severe reaction.
SubChapter: Compatibility and transfusion reactions

Q180. Answer: A

Explanation: Verification of correct recipient identifiers and crossmatch ensures product safety. Cryoprotectant and thawing checks apply only to frozen units. Chemotherapy date is clinically relevant but not infusion-specific.
SubChapter: Product verification and safety

Q181. Answer: B

Explanation: CAR-T therapy can trigger CRS, a systemic inflammatory response mediated by IL-6 and other cytokines; hallmark signs are fever and hemodynamic instability. Management includes tocilizumab and supportive care.
SubChapter: Cellular therapy complications

Q182. Answer: B

Explanation: Profound neutropenia heightens infection risk; protective isolation and meticulous hygiene prevent sepsis. Dietary liberalization or exercise can follow count recovery. Conditioning drugs are not stopped unless directed by the provider.
SubChapter: Conditioning complications – infection prevention

Q183. Answer: B
Explanation: The tingling is caused by citrate binding serum calcium during anticoagulation. Administering IV calcium gluconate corrects ionized calcium levels, alleviating symptoms rapidly. Stopping the collection interrupts therapy unnecessarily; increasing citrate would worsen hypocalcemia; warming provides comfort but not metabolic correction.
SubChapter: Apheresis – Metabolic Monitoring
Q184. Answer: B
Explanation: Busulfan neurotoxicity may progress to seizures; early reporting prompts adjustment of anticonvulsant prophylaxis (commonly levetiracetam). Observation alone risks escalation; hydration and rest offer little neurologic protection. Prompt intervention prevents irreversible complications and ensures treatment safety.
SubChapter: Chemotherapy Conditioning Toxicity
Q185. Answer: A
Explanation: Antipyretic, antihistamine, and corticosteroid pre-medications reduce fever, chills, and allergic responses to DMSO or donor plasma. Sedatives (B) may blunt monitoring; ondansetron (C) targets nausea alone; antibiotics (D) are unrelated to acute infusion reactions.
SubChapter: Infusion Pre-Medication Protocols
Q186. Answer: A
Explanation: Excessive heat damages cell membranes, leading to loss of viability and increased free hemoglobin. Immediate notification ensures quality control and replacement if necessary. Cooling abruptly causes osmotic shock; infusing compromised cells risks engraftment failure and hemolysis.
SubChapter: Product Thawing and Handling
Q187. Answer: B
Explanation: These are hallmark signs of acute hemolytic or allergic reaction. Stopping the infusion prevents further antigen exposure, maintaining IV access allows emergency medications. Diuretics or culture assessment follow after stabilization, not as first-line.
SubChapter: Acute Infusion Reactions
Q188. Answer: A
Explanation: Meticulous sterile dressing changes and hub decontamination are proven to reduce central-line infection risk. Routine systemic antibiotics encourage resistance; continuous heparin infusion increases bleeding risk; infrequent flushing promotes occlusion.
SubChapter: Apheresis – Access Care
Q189. Answer: B
Explanation: Mucosal care with bland rinses and analgesia maintains comfort and prevents infection in melphalan-induced mucositis. Carbonation irritates tissues; hard foods aggravate ulcers; fluid restriction worsens dehydration and healing delay.
SubChapter: Conditioning – Mucositis Management
Q190. Answer: B
Explanation: Product mislabeling constitutes a critical safety breach; infusion must be halted until verified by the cell-processing facility. Relabeling or proceeding breaches transfusion safety standards. Proper identity verification prevents catastrophic mismatched infusion.
SubChapter: Product Verification and Safety
Q191. Answer: A
Explanation: DLI can trigger cytokine surge from activated T-cells causing fever, rash, and malaise. GVHD typically develops days later; infection requires microbiologic confirmation; engraftment syndrome coincides with neutrophil recovery, not immediate post-infusion.
SubChapter: Cellular Therapy Complications
Q192. Answer: B

Explanation: Splenic rupture, though rare, is a known G-CSF complication; sudden LUQ pain warrants urgent imaging and discontinuation. Conservative measures delay diagnosis and risk hemorrhage. Early recognition prevents fatal outcomes.
SubChapter: Donor Safety and Mobilization

Q193. Answer: A

Explanation: Cyclophosphamide's metabolite acrolein causes bladder toxicity; mesna and hydration neutralize it. Failing to provide prophylaxis results in hemorrhagic cystitis. Antifungals and cranberry juice do not prevent chemical cystitis; antihypertensives are unrelated.
SubChapter: Conditioning – Toxicity Prevention

Q194. Answer: A

Explanation: Epinephrine rapidly reverses airway obstruction in anaphylaxis. Antihistamines and corticosteroids are secondary agents once airway is stabilized. Diuretics are irrelevant to allergic bronchospasm. Timely administration prevents respiratory collapse and death.
SubChapter: Acute Infusion Anaphylaxis Management

Q195. Answer: A

Explanation: A sudden fever may signal transfusion reaction or contamination; halting infusion limits exposure while assessment proceeds. Continuing may exacerbate systemic response. Antipyretics mask severity; delayed checks miss progression.
SubChapter: Infusion Reaction Response

Q196. Answer: B

Explanation: Inadequate CD34+ yield necessitates extended mobilization or additional collection. Infusing insufficient cells risks delayed engraftment. Adding plasma does not raise stem-cell count; storage alone is futile without meeting dose threshold.
SubChapter: Collection Yield Optimization

Q197. Answer: B

Explanation: TBI profoundly suppresses immunity; protective isolation safeguards the patient, not staff. Lead shielding protects staff during exposure but not afterward. Unrestricted visitation increases infection risk. Patient education reduces anxiety and improves cooperation.
SubChapter: Conditioning – Radiation Precautions

Q198. Answer: A

Explanation: Cardiovascular instability with bradycardia and hypertension signals DMSO toxicity. Immediate cessation and monitoring are essential. Sepsis presents with hypotension; delayed hemolysis occurs hours later. Recognition prevents severe cardiac events.
SubChapter: Cryoprotectant Reaction Management

Q199. Answer: A

Explanation: Controlled water-bath thawing evenly distributes heat and preserves bag integrity. Room-temperature thawing allows ice crystallization; opening the bag risks contamination; vigorous shaking damages cells. Precision ensures viable infusion product.
SubChapter: Product Handling and Safety

Q200. Answer: B

Explanation: Hypertension may accompany mild DMSO effects; reducing infusion rate and assessing symptoms prevent escalation. Discarding product wastes viable cells; diuretics unnecessary unless fluid overload exists. Ongoing monitoring ensures safety.
SubChapter: Infusion Monitoring

Questions (201-300)

Q201. Which laboratory result best confirms adequacy of hematopoietic stem-cell collection?

A. Platelet count > $50 \times 10^9/L$

B. CD34+ cell count ≥ 2×10^6 cells/kg

C. WBC > $5 \times 10^9/L$

D. Hematocrit > 30 %

Q202. During infusion, the patient develops chills and rigors without hypotension. Which nursing action is indicated?

A. Stop infusion and administer meperidine per protocol

B. Continue infusion and monitor vitals

C. Notify lab to test culture immediately

D. Increase infusion rate

Q203. A patient receiving a peripheral blood stem cell product complains of tightness in the throat and coughing during infusion. Which nursing action takes priority?

A. Stop infusion and administer oxygen

B. Slow infusion and reassess after 5 minutes

C. Give IV fluids rapidly

D. Notify lab to reissue product

Q204. During cell thawing, the nurse notices that the bag leaks at the tubing port. What is the safest next step?

A. Continue thawing and clamp above leak

B. Notify cell-processing lab and place bag in secondary sterile bag

C. Attempt to seal leak with tape and proceed

D. Discard immediately and request replacement

Q205. A patient becomes bradycardic and hypertensive during infusion of cryopreserved cells. What is the most likely cause?

A. Allergic transfusion reaction

B. DMSO toxicity

C. Citrate toxicity

D. Febrile reaction

Q206. A nurse notes air bubbles in the stem cell infusion tubing. What is the immediate nursing action?

A. Continue infusion; small bubbles are harmless

B. Stop infusion, clamp line, and remove air

C. Call provider before taking action

D. Increase infusion rate to clear the air

Q207. A patient experiences persistent nausea and vomiting after completing the conditioning regimen. What intervention should the nurse prioritize?

A. Encourage small frequent meals

B. Administer antiemetics and maintain hydration

C. Offer oral fluids only

D. Hold next chemotherapy dose

Q208. The nurse is preparing to collect peripheral stem cells and notes platelet count at $45 \times 10^9/L$. What is the best action?

A. Proceed as scheduled

B. Delay collection for one week

C. Notify the provider; may require platelet transfusion

D. Increase anticoagulant ratio during collection

Q209. A nurse observes patient complaints of tingling and cramps during apheresis. What concurrent monitoring parameter is essential?

A. Serum potassium
B. Ionized calcium level
C. Hemoglobin
D. Blood glucose

Q210. Which measure ensures accurate infusion of thawed cells?

A. Use of a blood filter
B. Gentle continuous agitation during infusion
C. Use of a controlled-rate syringe pump
D. Flushing with saline under pressure

Q211. A patient develops wheezing and hypotension during stem cell infusion despite premedication. Which medication should be administered immediately per protocol?

A. Epinephrine
B. Diphenhydramine
C. Hydrocortisone
D. Acetaminophen

Q212. Apheresis yield is below target after two collection days. What factor should the nurse assess first?

A. Donor hydration status
B. Machine calibration
C. G-CSF dose timing and compliance
D. Room temperature during collection

Q213. A patient receiving high-dose cyclophosphamide reports hematuria. What immediate nursing measure should be ensured?

A. Continue fluids and administer mesna
B. Reduce medication dose
C. Provide analgesics only
D. Restrict fluids to reduce bleeding

Q214. The nurse receives a product labeled "Haploidentical donor; volume 350 mL." What unique risk should be anticipated during infusion?

A. Acute hemolysis due to major ABO mismatch
B. Hypocalcemia from citrate
C. Nausea from DMSO
D. Delayed engraftment

Q215. A patient undergoing autologous transplant after BEAM conditioning reports fever and chills. Which potential cause must be ruled out first?

A. Neutropenic infection
B. Drug fever
C. Engraftment syndrome
D. Cytokine release

Q216. A donor experiences headache and bone pain after second G-CSF dose. What teaching point is most accurate?

A. Symptoms indicate allergic reaction
B. These are expected and manageable with non-opioid analgesics
C. G-CSF must be discontinued immediately
D. Use opioids to suppress marrow expansion pain

Q217. A nurse receives orders to infuse thawed product over 45 minutes, but patient develops rigors and hypertension after 10 minutes. What is the next nursing step?
A. Stop infusion temporarily and notify provider
B. Continue infusion but slow rate
C. Administer diuretics
D. Apply warm blankets only
Q218. During cell collection, calcium gluconate is administered via peripheral IV opposite the apheresis line. What is the rationale?
A. It prevents local irritation from citrate
B. It avoids interference with anticoagulant circuit
C. It maintains line patency
D. It improves venous return
Q219. A patient receiving total body irradiation expresses fear of radiation exposure to staff. What is the correct response?
A. "Staff exposure is minimal and controlled by distance and shielding."
B. "You will emit radiation for several days."
C. "Visitors must wear lead aprons for 24 hours."
D. "Exposure will make surfaces radioactive temporarily."
Q220. Apheresis collection ends early due to catheter clotting. Which prevention strategy should be emphasized for future sessions?
A. Heparinized saline flush between cycles
B. Increased flow pressure during collection
C. Avoiding line rest between cycles
D. Using smaller gauge catheters
Q221. A patient reports severe chills after infusion, with stable vital signs. What is the priority nursing action?
A. Stop infusion and administer meperidine
B. Continue and observe closely
C. Apply warm blankets only
D. Collect cultures immediately
Q222. During infusion, patient complains of metallic taste and headache. What is the likely cause?
A. Cryoprotectant DMSO effect
B. Hemolytic reaction
C. Hypocalcemia
D. Cytokine release
Q223. During marrow harvest, the donor develops light-headedness and pallor. What is the nurse's immediate priority?
A. Encourage deep breathing and continue
B. Administer IV fluids rapidly without assessment
C. Stop collection and place donor supine with legs elevated
D. Apply pressure to iliac site only
Q224. A patient undergoing reduced-intensity conditioning reports shortness of breath and non-productive cough. Chest x-ray shows diffuse infiltrates. Which complication should the nurse suspect?
A. Idiopathic pneumonia syndrome
B. Engraftment syndrome
C. Bacterial pneumonia
D. Pulmonary edema

Q225. During infusion of thawed allogeneic cells, patient develops severe headache and vomiting. Blood pressure 190/100 mm Hg. What is nurse's first action?

A. Stop infusion and assess for DMSO toxicity
B. Give antiemetic and continue
C. Notify lab for culture
D. Elevate head of bed and monitor

Q226. Apheresis line becomes occluded mid-collection. What is the safest first intervention?

A. Reposition patient and flush gently with saline
B. Apply suction to dislodge clot
C. Replace catheter immediately
D. Increase pump pressure

Q227. Following total-body irradiation, patient complains of parotid tenderness and dry mouth. What education should the nurse provide?

A. "Chew sugar-free gum and maintain oral hydration frequently."
B. "This indicates infection—antibiotics are required."
C. "Avoid any oral rinses."
D. "Stop all fluids until pain subsides."

Q228. Stem-cell infusion begins, and nurse notices product temperature still partially frozen. What should be done?

A. Warm bag under radiant heat
B. Continue slowly; thaw will finish in line
C. Stop infusion and complete thawing to 37 °C
D. Dilute with saline and proceed

Q229. A donor with small veins expresses concern about multiple sticks for apheresis. Which explanation is correct?

A. "Peripheral access may require two lines; a central catheter can be placed if needed."
B. "Only one vein is necessary for the entire procedure."
C. "We can draw blood intermittently instead."
D. "Apheresis uses needles smaller than routine draws."

Q230. A nurse detects rapid weight gain and right-upper-quadrant pain 10 days after conditioning. What is the likely cause?

A. Hepatic veno-occlusive disease
B. Acute GVHD
C. Engraftment syndrome
D. Cytokine release

Q231. While preparing infusion line, nurse connects product through a standard blood filter. What is the concern?

A. Stem cells may be trapped and lost within filter
B. Filter ensures sterility of infusion
C. It prevents large clots entering patient
D. It helps warm product gradually

Q232. A patient complains of burning sensation at IV site during infusion. What should nurse assess first?

A. Temperature of room
B. DMSO toxicity
C. Allergic reaction
D. Patency and infiltration of IV site

Q233. During marrow infusion, patient becomes febrile (39 °C) without hypotension. What is nurse's immediate response?
A. Stop infusion temporarily and notify provider
B. Continue infusion and record temperature
C. Give antipyretic only
D. Discard remaining product
Q234. Apheresis equipment alarm signals "high return pressure." What should nurse do first?
A. Check venous line for kinks or occlusion
B. Restart machine
C. Increase anticoagulant flow
D. Stop procedure permanently
Q235. Donor asks why G-CSF causes bone pain. The best response is:
A. "It stimulates marrow to produce and release more stem cells, expanding bone cavities."
B. "It increases calcium loss in bones."
C. "It inflames muscles, not bones."
D. "It alters blood pressure temporarily."
Q236. After thawing, the product bag develops a small puncture near tubing weld. What should nurse do?
A. Place in sterile overbag and inform processing lab immediately
B. Patch with sterile tape and continue
C. Discard quietly
D. Proceed to infusion to avoid delay
Q237. A patient develops urticaria and pruritus during infusion but remains hemodynamically stable. What is the initial nursing action?
A. Send blood for culture
B. Continue infusion and observe
C. Apply topical cream
D. Stop infusion temporarily and administer antihistamine
Q238. While preparing thaw bath, nurse uses uncalibrated thermometer reading 36 °C. Why is this a concern?
A. Inaccurate temperature may cause incomplete thaw or overheating, damaging cells
B. Slight differences are insignificant
C. Lower temperature ensures safety
D. Higher temperatures improve speed only
Q239. Patient receiving allogeneic transplant after conditioning develops epistaxis and petechiae. What lab value should nurse check first?
A. Platelet count
B. WBC count
C. Sodium
D. AST/ALT
Q240. During infusion, a nurse smells strong garlic odor in room. What does this signify?
A. Normal DMSO odor during infusion
B. Product contamination
C. Hemolysis
D. Reaction requiring immediate cessation
Q241. Patient with mismatched unrelated donor graft experiences dark urine during infusion. What should nurse do first?
A. Administer diphenhydramine

B. Give IV fluids immediately
C. Continue and document
D. Stop infusion and assess for hemolysis

Q242. A donor receiving plerixafor experiences mild diarrhea before collection. What should the nurse advise?
A. Maintain hydration and proceed as planned
B. Withhold drug dose
C. Replace plerixafor with G-CSF
D. Cancel collection

Q243. During apheresis, donor complains of numbness around lips and fingers. The nurse notes normal vital signs. What is the priority intervention?
A. Administer calcium gluconate slowly IV
B. Increase citrate infusion rate
C. Encourage deep breathing exercises
D. Pause collection for 10 minutes only

Q244. A patient receiving total body irradiation develops redness and blistering on the shoulders. What should the nurse do first?
A. Stop treatment and report possible radiation burn
B. Apply ice packs directly
C. Cover area with occlusive dressing
D. Encourage vigorous cleansing with soap

Q245. Apheresis donor develops nausea and abdominal cramping midway through procedure. Which action should nurse take?
A. Switch to heparin anticoagulation
B. Stop anticoagulant entirely
C. Continue and provide water
D. Decrease citrate flow rate and give calcium supplement

Q246. During infusion, patient suddenly complains of chest pain and dyspnea; O_2 saturation 88%. What is the immediate nursing action?
A. Stop infusion and administer oxygen
B. Administer acetaminophen
C. Increase infusion rate
D. Notify lab for contamination testing

Q247. A patient undergoing conditioning with busulfan reports dark urine and right-upper-quadrant tenderness. Which complication is suspected?
A. Hepatic veno-occlusive disease
B. Acute GVHD
C. Hemorrhagic cystitis
D. Cytokine release syndrome

Q248. Stem-cell bag leaks slightly during thawing. What is the safest immediate response?
A. Place in sterile over-bag and contact processing lab
B. Patch site with tape and continue infusion
C. Discard without notification
D. Wipe leak and proceed

Q249. Patient experiences fever and rigors 15 minutes into infusion. What should the nurse do first?
A. Increase infusion rate
B. Administer acetaminophen and continue
C. Collect cultures before stopping

D. Stop infusion and assess for reaction

Q250. Apheresis flow stops abruptly. Machine displays "access pressure low." What should nurse assess first?

A. Catheter kinking or patient position
B. Anticoagulant ratio
C. Hemoglobin level
D. Calcium infusion rate

Q251. After cyclophosphamide conditioning, patient develops hematuria. Which preventive therapy may have been missed?

A. Mesna and vigorous hydration
B. Allopurinol
C. Levofloxacin
D. Ondansetron

Q252. Donor reports severe bone pain on day 4 of G-CSF mobilization. What teaching should nurse reinforce?

A. Use NSAIDs or acetaminophen; pain resolves after collection
B. Stop G-CSF immediately
C. Pain indicates infection
D. Massage affected areas vigorously

Q253. During thawing, nurse notes persistent ice crystals. What is the correct next action?

A. Shake vigorously
B. Proceed immediately to infusion
C. Raise bath temperature to 45 °C
D. Continue warming until fully clear at 37 °C

Q254. A patient receiving mismatched unrelated donor graft develops back pain and red urine mid-infusion. What is the priority action?

A. Stop infusion; suspect hemolytic transfusion reaction
B. Continue at slower rate
C. Flush line with saline and continue
D. Notify housekeeping for specimen disposal

Q255. Apheresis donor develops tingling after prolonged procedure; calcium infusion ongoing. What additional intervention is indicated?

A. Reassess rate and provide oral calcium supplement
B. Stop citrate infusion
C. Ignore; normal finding
D. Increase citrate to maintain anticoagulation

Q256. During infusion, BP rises and patient complains of nausea. Which complication should nurse consider?

A. DMSO toxicity
B. Sepsis
C. Engraftment syndrome
D. Hemorrhagic cystitis

Q257. A patient receiving fresh (non-cryopreserved) stem cells asks why no thawing is required. Best explanation?

A. "Fresh products are collected and infused immediately without freezing."
B. "Thawing would activate cells prematurely."
C. "Freezing destroys stem cells."
D. "The cells are stored only at room temperature."

Q258. During conditioning, patient develops oral ulcers and difficulty swallowing. What priority intervention prevents further complications?
A. Restrict fluids
B. Encourage acidic juices
C. Continue conditioning unaltered
D. Implement bland rinses, pain control, and nutritional support
Q259. During cell collection, donor complains of tingling and mild cramps despite calcium infusion. Which assessment is essential?
A. Ionized calcium level
B. Potassium level
C. Hematocrit
D. Temperature
Q260. Patient complains of garlic-like breath odor during infusion. What should nurse explain?
A. It results from DMSO excretion through lungs and is temporary
B. It indicates infection
C. It is due to blood contamination
D. It signals reaction requiring stopping infusion
Q261. Donor experiences dizziness and diaphoresis at end of collection. BP 80/50 mm Hg. What is nurse's first action?
A. Stop procedure, lower head, elevate legs
B. Give caffeine beverage
C. Apply cool compress
D. Ask donor to stand and stretch
Q262. A nurse observes cloudy stem-cell product before infusion. What should be done?
A. Filter through leukocyte filter
B. Infuse under close observation
C. Hold infusion and notify processing lab for evaluation
D. Warm to dissolve clumps
Q263. A patient receiving thawed stem-cell product suddenly becomes flushed with chest tightness and anxiety. Which action should the nurse take first?
A. Stop the infusion and maintain IV access with normal saline
B. Administer diphenhydramine immediately
C. Reassure the patient and slow the infusion
D. Apply cool compresses to the chest
Q264. Apheresis operator reports frequent clot alarms. Which factor should the nurse verify first?
A. Anticoagulant flow rate
B. Donor platelet count
C. Machine software version
D. Calcium infusion concentration
Q265. After melphalan conditioning, the patient reports severe mouth pain and inability to swallow. What intervention best supports continued therapy?
A. Initiate parenteral nutrition and analgesic mouth rinses
B. Continue oral intake despite pain
C. Provide only ice chips
D. Delay transplant until mucosa heals
Q266. While infusing cells, the nurse observes patient shivering violently without hypotension. What should be done?
A. Continue at slower rate

B. Apply warm blankets only
C. Stop infusion and administer meperidine per protocol
D. Start broad-spectrum antibiotics

Q267. Apheresis donor exhibits tingling and muscle cramps despite IV calcium. Which step optimizes management?
A. Check ionized calcium and adjust infusion rate
B. Stop collection immediately
C. Increase citrate dose
D. Offer oral fluids

Q268. The nurse receives a product labeled with the wrong birth date but correct name. What should be done?
A. Hold infusion and verify with cell-processing lab
B. Proceed if medical record number matches
C. Relabel bag at bedside
D. Ask another nurse to confirm and continue

Q269. A patient reports dizziness and metallic taste immediately after start of infusion. BP 170/95 mm Hg. What is likely cause?
A. DMSO toxicity causing transient hypertension
B. Sepsis from contamination
C. Citrate toxicity
D. Engraftment syndrome

Q270. During donor apheresis, venous line suddenly becomes pale and sluggish. What should nurse do?
A. Flush with heparin bolus
B. Increase pump speed
C. Restart new access immediately
D. Reposition arm and verify patency

Q271. Patient receiving high-dose busulfan reports seizures despite prophylaxis. Which action should nurse anticipate?
A. Increase anticonvulsant dose and monitor levels
B. Discontinue busulfan immediately
C. Provide cooling blanket
D. Administer calcium

Q272. A nurse notices mild clumping in thawed stem-cell product. What step ensures patient safety?
A. Notify lab for viability testing before infusion
B. Filter through standard blood filter
C. Warm rapidly to 45 °C
D. Infuse immediately to avoid waste

Q273. A patient experiences burning at IV site during infusion. What is nurse's immediate response?
A. Stop infusion and assess for infiltration
B. Apply warm compress and continue
C. Administer diphenhydramine
D. Flush vigorously

Q274. Following infusion, patient develops oliguria and rising creatinine. What complication is suspected?
A. Tumor lysis
B. Engraftment syndrome
C. Veno-occlusive disease

D. Hemolysis-induced acute kidney injury

Q275. Donor with central catheter reports mild erythema at insertion site. What should nurse do?

A. Assess for infection and apply aseptic dressing
B. Remove line immediately
C. Ignore unless febrile
D. Flush with antibiotic solution

Q276. Patient reports severe nausea during stem-cell infusion. Which is the most appropriate immediate intervention?

A. Administer prescribed antiemetic and slow infusion rate
B. Stop infusion permanently
C. Encourage deep breathing
D. Offer ice chips

Q277. Apheresis donor exhibits anxiety and hyperventilation early in procedure. What should nurse do?

A. Provide reassurance and coach slow breathing
B. Stop procedure immediately
C. Increase citrate flow
D. Administer sedative without evaluation

Q278. During conditioning, patient's WBC = 0.2×10^9/L. Which nursing action has highest priority?

A. Continue fresh fruit intake
B. Encourage group physical therapy
C. Limit oral care
D. Implement neutropenic precautions and monitor temperature

Q279. While preparing thaw bath, water temperature reads 34 °C. What should nurse do?

A. Adjust to 37 °C before inserting product
B. Proceed; difference insignificant
C. Raise temperature to 40 °C
D. Add cold water after thawing

Q280. During collection, donor complains of tingling despite adequate calcium infusion. BP drops to 85/55 mm Hg. What complication should be suspected?

A. Vasovagal episode from volume depletion
B. Citrate toxicity
C. Sepsis
D. Allergic reaction

Q281. A nurse preparing cryopreserved cells notes bag labeled "Store ≤ −150 °C." What is the rationale?

A. Ultra-low storage prevents ice-crystal formation preserving viability
B. It allows bacteria to be destroyed
C. It ensures product remains sterile after thawing
D. It accelerates post-thaw engraftment

Q282. Patient develops fever 4 hours after infusion completion. Which cause must nurse rule out first?

A. GVHD
B. Engraftment syndrome
C. Infusion-related contamination or sepsis
D. Cytokine release

Q283. A patient develops flushing and chest pressure five minutes into infusion. What should the nurse do first?

A. Stop infusion now
B. Slow infusion rate
C. Give fluids fast
D. Call provider now

Q284. Apheresis donor reports tingling fingers during collection. What is the best action?
A. Give IV calcium
B. Stop procedure
C. Offer snack food
D. Raise arm height

Q285. Patient complains of metallic taste mid-infusion. What should nurse explain?
A. Normal DMSO effect
B. Drug error sign
C. Infection signal
D. Reaction onset

Q286. Stem-cell bag shows small leak during thawing. What should nurse do?
A. Discard quietly
B. Wipe and use
C. Seal and notify
D. Delay without report

Q287. Patient receiving TBI reports sore mouth after day 2. What is best teaching?
A. Use bland rinse
B. Brush with salt
C. Chew hard food
D. Drink citrus juice

Q288. During infusion, BP rises to 180/100 mm Hg. Patient feels dizzy. Next step?
A. Pause infusion
B. Give antacid
C. Ignore BP
D. Continue slow

Q289. Apheresis alarm shows "low return pressure." Nurse should first:
A. Check line kink
B. Add anticoag
C. Restart device
D. Stop process

Q290. Patient has fever and chills after infusion. Nurse should:
A. Wait for rounds
B. Give acetamin
C. Continue slow
D. Stop and assess

Q291. Donor complains of pain at catheter site. Nurse should:
A. Inspect and clean
B. Apply heat pad
C. Continue run
D. Change tape

Q292. During conditioning, patient develops confusion. What should nurse check first?
A. Serum sodium
B. WBC count
C. ALT/AST

D. Platelet count

Q293. While infusing, nurse smells garlic odor. Appropriate action?

A. Reassure patient
B. Stop infusion
C. Vent room air
D. Add filter line

Q294. Patient's urine becomes red during infusion. First step?

A. Reassure only
B. Continue slow
C. Offer fluids
D. Stop and check

Q295. Apheresis donor feels dizzy near end of procedure. What should nurse do?

A. Lower head flat
B. Stop machine
C. Give coffee drink
D. Raise arms high

Q296. During thawing, bath reads 34 °C. Nurse should:

A. Adjust to 37 °C
B. Add more bags
C. Proceed anyway
D. Raise to 45 °C

Q297. Patient develops cough and dyspnea post-infusion. What is priority?

A. Assess oxygen and notify
B. Give cough syrup
C. Continue infusion
D. Encourage walking

Q298. During apheresis, donor reports cold feeling. Nurse should:

A. Increase speed
B. Stop collection
C. Provide blanket
D. Give diuretic

Q299. After cyclophosphamide, patient develops gross hematuria. Nurse anticipates:

A. Mesna therapy
B. Morphine dose
C. Antibiotic change
D. Diet adjust

Q300. Infusion line disconnects briefly. What should nurse do?

A. Replace set aseptically
B. Reconnect quickly
C. Flush and continue
D. Tape connection

Answer key and Explanation (201-300)

Q201. Answer: B

Explanation: Successful engraftment requires at least 2 × 10^6 CD34+ cells/kg; lower counts prolong recovery. Platelet or WBC counts are nonspecific. Monitoring this parameter guides collection end-points and transplant readiness.

SubChapter: Collection Adequacy Criteria

Q202. Answer: A

Explanation: Rigors signify febrile non-hemolytic reaction; meperidine alleviates rigors while halting infusion prevents progression. Continuing may exacerbate symptoms; culture testing follows if contamination suspected. Prompt action ensures patient safety.

SubChapter: Infusion Reaction Management

Q203. Answer: A

Explanation: Sudden throat tightness and cough indicate airway involvement in an acute allergic or anaphylactoid reaction, possibly due to donor plasma or DMSO. Stopping infusion and administering oxygen ensures airway protection and prepares for emergency medication. Delaying action or continuing infusion risks respiratory compromise.

SubChapter: Infusion Complication – Airway Reaction

Q204. Answer: B

Explanation: Leaks compromise sterility; notifying the lab ensures documentation and decision on salvage or replacement. Placing the unit in a sterile overbag prevents environmental contamination during transport. Continuing thawing or patching breaches protocol, and discarding without evaluation wastes viable product.

SubChapter: Product Handling & Contamination Control

Q205. Answer: B

Explanation: DMSO toxicity manifests with cardiovascular instability such as hypertension, bradycardia, and chest pressure. Recognition is essential to prevent arrhythmia or cardiac arrest. Citrate toxicity presents as hypocalcemia and tetany; febrile reactions cause chills and fever, not blood pressure spikes.

SubChapter: Cryoprotectant-Related Reactions

Q206. Answer: B

Explanation: Air in central lines poses a risk of embolism. Stopping infusion and clearing air safely prevents cardiorespiratory compromise. Increasing rate or continuing could introduce air into circulation, potentially fatal. Immediate nurse-led intervention is within safe practice guidelines.

SubChapter: Infusion Technique Safety

Q207. Answer: B

Explanation: Conditioning-related gastrointestinal toxicity requires proactive antiemetic management and hydration to prevent dehydration and electrolyte imbalance. Nutritional adjustments assist later. Chemotherapy doses are managed by providers, not nursing independently.

SubChapter: Conditioning Supportive Care

Q208. Answer: C

Explanation: Low platelet count heightens bleeding risk during apheresis; provider notification ensures appropriate transfusion support before collection. Proceeding unsafely risks hemorrhage; delaying a full week may interrupt mobilization timing; altering anticoagulant does not resolve thrombocytopenia.

SubChapter: Collection Safety Parameters

Q209. Answer: B

Explanation: Citrate chelates calcium during apheresis; monitoring ionized calcium identifies hypocalcemia before severe symptoms develop. Potassium or glucose are not directly altered by citrate use. Tracking this value guides IV calcium supplementation safely.

SubChapter: Apheresis – Citrate Monitoring

Q210. Answer: B
Explanation: Gentle agitation prevents cell sedimentation and ensures even delivery. Blood filters trap stem cells; syringe pumps exert excessive pressure, risking cell lysis; high-pressure saline flushes damage cells. Proper technique safeguards engraftment potential.
SubChapter: Infusion Technique Optimization
Q211. Answer: A
Explanation: Epinephrine is life-saving in anaphylaxis, reversing bronchospasm and hypotension through vasoconstriction and bronchodilation. Other agents act slower and serve adjunct roles. Prompt use prevents cardiac arrest.
SubChapter: Acute Anaphylaxis Response
Q212. Answer: C
Explanation: Poor mobilization often results from suboptimal G-CSF adherence or timing. Verifying administration ensures effective CD34+ release. Hydration or environmental factors have lesser impact. Calibration issues are rare but secondary considerations.
SubChapter: Collection Optimization Factors
Q213. Answer: A
Explanation: Mesna neutralizes toxic metabolites in urine, preventing hemorrhagic cystitis; continuous hydration dilutes irritants. Dose adjustment or restriction decisions belong to the provider; symptom management alone neglects cause control.
SubChapter: Conditioning Toxicity Prevention
Q214. Answer: A
Explanation: Haploidentical grafts often have partial ABO incompatibility, risking intravascular hemolysis. Vigilant monitoring for hemoglobinuria, back pain, and hypotension is essential. Other effects may occur but hemolysis is the distinct risk requiring readiness for emergency management.
SubChapter: Compatibility Management
Q215. Answer: A
Explanation: During aplasia, any fever is presumed infectious until proven otherwise. Prompt cultures and empiric antibiotics reduce sepsis mortality. Other causes remain secondary until infection is excluded.
SubChapter: Post-Conditioning Infection Risk
Q216. Answer: B
Explanation: G-CSF stimulates marrow activity causing transient bone pain; NSAIDs or acetaminophen usually suffice. Education reassures donor safety. Stopping unnecessarily compromises mobilization. True allergic reactions are rare and present differently.
SubChapter: Donor Mobilization Effects
Q217. Answer: A
Explanation: Stopping infusion prevents escalation of suspected reaction and allows provider intervention with antihistamines or steroids. Slowing rate alone can worsen cumulative exposure. Comfort measures are supportive but not definitive management.
SubChapter: Infusion Reaction Protocols
Q218. Answer: B
Explanation: Administering calcium separately prevents neutralization of citrate anticoagulant within the collection circuit, ensuring continuous flow and preventing clot formation. Same-line infusion would compromise collection efficiency.
SubChapter: Apheresis Technique
Q219. Answer: A

Explanation: TBI delivers external radiation; patients are not radioactive afterward. Education alleviates fear and fosters cooperation. Other statements perpetuate myths and anxiety. Proper information reinforces trust and compliance with therapy.
SubChapter: Conditioning – Radiation Education

Q220. Answer: A

Explanation: Regular heparinized saline flushes prevent fibrin formation and catheter occlusion. Excessive pressure or smaller catheters exacerbate mechanical stress. Periodic line rest does not affect clot formation directly.
SubChapter: Apheresis Line Maintenance

Q221. Answer: A

Explanation: Rigors without hypotension indicate febrile non-hemolytic reaction; meperidine provides rapid relief and prevents worsening. Cultures may follow if infection suspected, but symptomatic control and safety take precedence. Continuing infusion risks escalation.
SubChapter: Infusion Reaction – Rigors

Q222. Answer: A

Explanation: DMSO imparts transient metallic or garlic-like taste and mild headache due to volatility. Reassurance and slow infusion alleviate discomfort. These symptoms are benign compared to severe DMSO toxicity, which includes cardiovascular instability.
SubChapter: Cryopreserved Product Effects

Q223. Answer: C

Explanation: Acute vasovagal or volume-related hypotension requires prompt cessation, positioning for perfusion, and assessment before resuming. Rapid fluids may worsen discomfort without evaluation. Continuing procedure risks collapse. Local pressure alone ignores systemic cause and delays recovery.
SubChapter: Collection Safety – Donor Stability

Q224. Answer: A

Explanation: Idiopathic pneumonia syndrome occurs after conditioning from cytokine-mediated alveolar damage, independent of infection. Prompt identification enables corticosteroid therapy. Infection presents with fevers; edema manifests with volume overload signs. Recognition differentiates non-infectious pulmonary toxicity early.
SubChapter: Conditioning-Related Pulmonary Toxicity

Q225. Answer: A

Explanation: Hypertension and neurologic symptoms during infusion suggest DMSO toxicity; stopping infusion prevents progression to hypertensive crisis or seizure. Supportive medications follow once stable. Culture and positioning do not address acute cause.
SubChapter: Infusion Complication – Cryoprotectant Toxicity

Q226. Answer: A

Explanation: Most occlusions stem from positional or fibrin issues; gentle flush under sterile conditions restores flow safely. Forcing pressure or suction may rupture the line or dislodge thrombi. Catheter replacement follows persistent blockage.
SubChapter: Apheresis Line Troubleshooting

Q227. Answer: A

Explanation: Radiation damages salivary glands causing xerostomia; salivary stimulation and hydration reduce mucosal injury and infection risk. Antibiotics are indicated only if infection confirmed; avoiding rinses worsens dryness.
SubChapter: Conditioning Side-Effect Management

Q228. Answer: C

Explanation: Infusing partially frozen product causes cellular rupture and occlusion in microvasculature. Full thaw in controlled 37 °C water bath preserves viability. Radiant heat overheats locally; saline dilution alters osmolarity.
SubChapter: Product Thaw Quality Control
Q229. Answer: A
Explanation: Continuous apheresis requires simultaneous draw and return lines; difficult access may necessitate central catheter. Honesty and education build trust. Minimizing disclosure misleads donor and risks collection delays.
SubChapter: Donor Preparation and Education
Q230. Answer: A
Explanation: VOD arises from hepatic endothelial injury by alkylating agents, producing hepatomegaly, ascites, and weight gain. Early identification allows defibrotide or supportive therapy. GVHD manifests later; engraftment and CRS have distinct timing and findings.
SubChapter: Conditioning Toxicity – Hepatic
Q231. Answer: A
Explanation: Hematopoietic stem cells adhere to standard filters, reducing viable cell dose and delaying engraftment. Specialized tubing without filter is required. Sterility and clot prevention are ensured during processing, not via transfusion filters.
SubChapter: Infusion Equipment Standards
Q232. Answer: D
Explanation: Local pain often indicates infiltration or extravasation; verifying patency prevents tissue injury and cell loss. Systemic reactions cause generalized symptoms rather than local burning. Room temperature is irrelevant.
SubChapter: Infusion Site Assessment
Q233. Answer: A
Explanation: Even isolated fever can signal infusion reaction or contamination; pausing allows assessment and cultures. Continuing may worsen reaction. Discarding prematurely wastes irreplaceable cells.
SubChapter: Infusion Reaction – Fever Response
Q234. Answer: A
Explanation: Elevated return pressure commonly results from tubing kink or positional issue; correction restores flow. Restarting or altering anticoagulant doesn't fix mechanical cause. Stopping permanently is unnecessary unless unresolved.
SubChapter: Apheresis Troubleshooting
Q235. Answer: A
Explanation: G-CSF accelerates myelopoiesis, expanding intramedullary pressure and causing transient bone discomfort, particularly in pelvis and sternum. Education normalizes expectations and reassures safety. Other explanations are incorrect physiologically.
SubChapter: Donor Education – Mobilization Effects
Q236. Answer: A
Explanation: Even small breaches compromise sterility; secure overbag prevents leakage and contamination until lab verifies usability. Taping or infusing damaged bags violates safety standards and risks septic infusion.
SubChapter: Product Integrity Management
Q237. Answer: D
Explanation: Mild allergic reactions respond to antihistamines; pausing prevents escalation. Continuing can lead to anaphylaxis. Topical measures insufficient. Cultures apply to suspected infection, not allergy.
SubChapter: Allergic Reaction Management

Q238. Answer: A
Explanation: Accurate 37 °C calibration ensures cell membrane stability; deviations cause ice retention or heat shock, reducing viability. Reliability of equipment is crucial for consistent engraftment outcomes.
SubChapter: Equipment Calibration & Quality Assurance
Q239. Answer: A
Explanation: Thrombocytopenia due to marrow ablation is common; assessing platelet level directs transfusion support. White-cell counts or liver enzymes do not explain bleeding manifestations directly. Early replacement prevents hemorrhage complications.
SubChapter: Conditioning Hematologic Effects
Q240. Answer: A
Explanation: Volatile DMSO vaporizes through patient's breath, creating distinct garlic odor; benign but notable. Staff awareness prevents alarm. Contamination or hemolysis present differently with color or clinical symptoms.
SubChapter: Cryoprotectant Education
Q241. Answer: D
Explanation: Dark urine suggests hemoglobinuria from incompatible plasma; stopping infusion prevents renal damage. Supportive fluids follow after confirmation. Continuing allows progression to shock.
SubChapter: Compatibility – Hemolytic Reaction
Q242. Answer: A
Explanation: Plerixafor's GI side effects are transient; hydration prevents volume depletion and does not affect mobilization efficiency. Stopping or substituting medication disrupts schedule unnecessarily.
SubChapter: Mobilization Agent Side Effect Management
Q243. Answer: A
Explanation: Hypocalcemia from citrate anticoagulant causes perioral tingling and paresthesias. Intravenous calcium reverses symptoms and prevents progression to tetany or arrhythmia. Increasing citrate worsens the deficit; breathing exercises are ineffective; short pauses may not restore balance without supplementation.
SubChapter: Collection Metabolic Complications
Q244. Answer: A
Explanation: Radiation burns indicate excessive local dose or skin sensitivity; halting therapy and medical review prevent deeper injury. Ice and harsh cleaning aggravate damage; occlusive dressings trap heat. Prompt documentation ensures safety and dose verification.
SubChapter: Conditioning – Radiation Toxicity
Q245. Answer: D
Explanation: Citrate toxicity manifests with GI and neuromuscular symptoms. Adjusting flow rate and calcium replacement alleviates discomfort safely. Stopping anticoagulation risks clotting; switching anticoagulants mid-procedure is not standard. Hydration alone provides minimal relief.
SubChapter: Apheresis – Citrate Management
Q246. Answer: A
Explanation: Sudden respiratory distress suggests acute infusion reaction or pulmonary embolic event; stopping infusion halts antigen exposure, oxygen improves tissue perfusion. Analgesics mask symptoms; increasing rate exacerbates hypoxia. Contamination testing follows stabilization.
SubChapter: Infusion Reaction – Respiratory
Q247. Answer: A
Explanation: Busulfan causes sinusoidal endothelial injury leading to hepatic obstruction, ascites, and jaundice. Early recognition allows initiation of defibrotide and supportive management. GVHD appears later; cystitis is bladder-related; CRS occurs with cell therapies, not chemotherapy conditioning.
SubChapter: Conditioning Hepatic Toxicity

Q248. Answer: A
Explanation: Any compromise of bag sterility mandates secure containment and laboratory evaluation to maintain product integrity. Proceeding risks contamination and sepsis; patching violates asepsis. Communication ensures traceability and replacement authorization.
SubChapter: Product Integrity and Safety
Q249. Answer: D
Explanation: Early fever can indicate febrile non-hemolytic or allergic reaction; pausing limits exposure and allows evaluation. Continuing may worsen systemic effects. Cultures are secondary once reaction ruled out.
SubChapter: Infusion Reaction Assessment
Q250. Answer: A
Explanation: Mechanical obstruction from patient movement or tubing kink commonly causes low access pressure. Checking and correcting position restores flow safely. Chemical parameters do not affect pressure directly.
SubChapter: Apheresis Equipment Troubleshooting
Q251. Answer: A
Explanation: Mesna binds acrolein, cyclophosphamide's toxic metabolite, preventing hemorrhagic cystitis. Hydration flushes irritants. Allopurinol prevents tumor lysis, not bladder toxicity; antibiotics and antiemetics are unrelated.
SubChapter: Conditioning – Urotoxicity Prevention
Q252. Answer: A
Explanation: Bone pain is common due to marrow expansion; mild analgesics effectively control symptoms. It resolves post-collection. Discontinuing drug reduces stem-cell yield; vigorous massage risks trauma; infection signs differ.
SubChapter: Donor Mobilization Education
Q253. Answer: D
Explanation: Complete thawing at 37 °C ensures all cells are viable; residual ice damages membranes. Higher temperatures or agitation destroy cells. Precision preserves engraftment potential.
SubChapter: Product Thaw Technique
Q254. Answer: A
Explanation: Back pain and hemoglobinuria indicate acute hemolysis from ABO incompatibility. Immediate cessation prevents shock and renal failure. Supportive care and labs follow. Slowing or flushing worsens exposure.
SubChapter: Compatibility – Transfusion Reaction
Q255. Answer: A
Explanation: Persistent symptoms suggest inadequate replacement; oral calcium complements IV supply safely. Stopping anticoagulant risks clotting; increasing citrate aggravates imbalance. Monitoring ensures donor comfort and safety.
SubChapter: Apheresis Metabolic Support
Q256. Answer: A
Explanation: Hypertension with nausea and odor indicates moderate DMSO effect. Slowing infusion and supportive monitoring suffice. Sepsis presents with hypotension; engraftment syndrome occurs later post-transplant.
SubChapter: Cryoprotectant Reactions
Q257. Answer: A
Explanation: Fresh collections remain liquid and are infused soon after harvest; cryopreservation applies only for storage or transport. Explaining process improves understanding and trust. Other statements misrepresent lab procedures.

SubChapter: Product Processing Education

Q258. Answer: D

Explanation: Mucositis care maintains oral integrity, reduces infection risk, and preserves nutrition. Acidic beverages irritate tissues; withholding hydration worsens dehydration. Coordinated symptom management supports therapy tolerance.

SubChapter: Conditioning Toxicity – Mucositis

Q259. Answer: A

Explanation: Measuring ionized calcium confirms effectiveness of replacement and guides adjustment. Total serum calcium may be misleading; potassium or hematocrit are unrelated to citrate effects.

SubChapter: Collection Monitoring

Q260. Answer: A

Explanation: DMSO volatilizes via pulmonary route, producing characteristic odor for up to 48 hours. Reassurance normalizes expectation and prevents anxiety. It is benign, not infectious.

SubChapter: Cryoprotectant Education

Q261. Answer: A

Explanation: Hypotension from volume loss or vasovagal episode requires Trendelenburg positioning and rest to restore circulation. Caffeine and movement aggravate collapse. Early recognition prevents injury.

SubChapter: Donor Safety – Hypotension

Q262. Answer: C

Explanation: Cloudiness may signify contamination or cellular lysis; infusion must be withheld until sterility and viability confirmed. Filtering removes viable cells; heating worsens damage. Strict adherence ensures patient safety and product integrity.

SubChapter: Product Quality Control

Q263. Answer: A

Explanation: Acute allergic or anaphylactoid reactions present with flushing, chest pressure, and anxiety. The priority is stopping infusion to halt antigen exposure while maintaining IV access for emergency drugs and fluids. Symptom treatment follows. Cooling and reassurance alone delay life-saving interventions.

SubChapter: Infusion Reaction – Immediate Response

Q264. Answer: A

Explanation: Inadequate citrate anticoagulation promotes circuit clotting. Verifying anticoagulant flow prevents yield loss and line occlusion. Platelet count or software issues rarely cause alarms; calcium supplementation does not affect anticoagulation efficacy.

SubChapter: Collection Process – Anticoagulation Control

Q265. Answer: A

Explanation: Severe mucositis requires aggressive symptom control and nutrition maintenance. Parenteral nutrition prevents catabolism, and analgesic rinses enable comfort. Delaying transplant risks disease progression. Limiting intake or relying on ice chips worsens dehydration and malnutrition.

SubChapter: Conditioning Toxicity – Mucositis Management

Q266. Answer: C

Explanation: Rigors signify febrile non-hemolytic or mild allergic reaction; halting infusion limits exposure, and meperidine provides rapid relief. Warmth aids comfort but not cause. Antibiotics apply if infection suspected after evaluation. Continuing may escalate to severe reaction.

SubChapter: Infusion Reaction – Rigors

Q267. Answer: A

Explanation: Ongoing symptoms indicate inadequate calcium replacement; verifying ionized calcium guides proper dosing. Stopping collection prematurely reduces yield unnecessarily. Increasing citrate aggravates hypocalcemia; oral hydration alone is insufficient correction.
SubChapter: Collection – Metabolic Monitoring

Q268. Answer: A

Explanation: Any labeling discrepancy constitutes potential mismatch; infusion must stop until verified by the issuing laboratory. Proceeding without verification risks serious transfusion error. Relabeling independently violates regulatory standards.
SubChapter: Product Verification & Safety

Q269. Answer: A

Explanation: DMSO triggers sympathetic stimulation, producing hypertension and metallic taste early in infusion. Usually self-limited but requires rate adjustment and observation. Sepsis presents later with hypotension; citrate reactions occur during collection, not infusion.
SubChapter: Cryoprotectant Reactions

Q270. Answer: D

Explanation: Positional changes frequently obstruct flow; adjusting limb position restores access. Increasing pressure may collapse vein. Starting new line or heparin bolus is premature without assessment.
SubChapter: Apheresis Line Management

Q271. Answer: A

Explanation: Busulfan lowers seizure threshold; adjusting prophylactic medication prevents recurrence while continuing regimen safely under medical direction. Stopping therapy prematurely disrupts conditioning. Cooling and calcium offer no neurologic benefit.
SubChapter: Conditioning Neurotoxicity Management

Q272. Answer: A

Explanation: Clumping may indicate membrane rupture or thawing error; lab confirmation prevents infusion of non-viable cells or aggregates causing emboli. Filters trap stem cells; overheating destroys viability.
SubChapter: Product Quality Control

Q273. Answer: A

Explanation: Local pain suggests infiltration; prompt assessment prevents tissue necrosis and cell loss. Continuing or flushing under pressure may worsen extravasation. Systemic drugs are irrelevant unless reaction proven.
SubChapter: Infusion Site Assessment

Q274. Answer: D

Explanation: Hemoglobinuria from hemolytic reaction or damaged product can precipitate renal injury. Adequate hydration and monitoring are essential. Engraftment and VOD affect different organs; tumor lysis occurs with cytotoxic therapy, not infusion.
SubChapter: Infusion Complications – Renal Effects

Q275. Answer: A

Explanation: Early redness warrants evaluation for infection or irritation; cleansing and dressing replacement prevent progression. Removal reserved for confirmed infection. Prophylactic antibiotic flushes are not evidence-based.
SubChapter: Apheresis Access Care

Q276. Answer: A

Explanation: Nausea is common DMSO side effect; antiemetics and rate adjustment relieve symptoms while maintaining therapy. Permanent cessation unnecessary unless severe toxicity develops. Non-pharmacologic measures provide limited relief alone.

SubChapter: Cryoprotectant Symptom Management

Q277. Answer: A

Explanation: Anxiety may mimic hypocalcemia; calm coaching stabilizes breathing and improves tolerance. Stopping or altering anticoagulation is unnecessary. Sedatives are last resort after non-pharmacologic techniques fail.

SubChapter: Donor Comfort & Psychological Support

Q278. Answer: D

Explanation: Profound neutropenia requires strict infection prevention—hand hygiene, protective isolation, and temperature monitoring for sepsis. Physical contact and unwashed foods pose infection risks. Vigilance during aplasia prevents fatal infections.

SubChapter: Conditioning – Infection Prevention

Q279. Answer: A

Explanation: Optimal 37 °C ensures uniform thawing and cell viability. Lower temperature prolongs exposure to ice crystals damaging membranes. Overheating or inconsistent control reduces engraftment potential.

SubChapter: Equipment Calibration – Thaw Process

Q280. Answer: A

Explanation: Hypotension and dizziness without tetany indicate vasovagal response due to anxiety or fluid shifts. Trendelenburg positioning and reassurance restore stability. Citrate toxicity typically elevates BP and causes paresthesias without hypotension.

SubChapter: Donor Safety – Vasovagal Management

Q281. Answer: A

Explanation: Cryogenic temperatures below glass transition prevent recrystallization and maintain cell structure. Sterility and engraftment depend on asepsis and biologic factors, not temperature alone. Understanding this reinforces importance of cold-chain management.

SubChapter: Product Storage Standards

Q282. Answer: C

Explanation: Fever soon after infusion may signal bacterial contamination; cultures and empiric antibiotics are urgent. Engraftment or GVHD occur days later. Rapid investigation preserves patient safety and infection control standards.

SubChapter: Post-Infusion Complications – Infection

Q283. Answer: A

Explanation: Flushing and chest pressure signal acute hypersensitivity or DMSO toxicity. Immediate cessation halts antigen exposure while maintaining IV access for emergency medications. Delay or rate adjustment risks airway compromise and cardiovascular instability.

SubChapter: Infusion Reaction Management

Q284. Answer: A

Explanation: Tingling reflects citrate-induced hypocalcemia. Administering IV calcium promptly prevents progression to muscle spasms or arrhythmia. Stopping collection unnecessarily reduces yield; snacks or position change do not correct electrolyte deficit.

SubChapter: Collection Metabolic Care

Q285. Answer: A

Explanation: Dimethyl sulfoxide produces a transient metallic or garlic-like taste as it volatilizes. It is harmless and expected. Misinterpreting as infection or drug error causes undue concern; reassurance maintains compliance.

SubChapter: Cryoprotectant Education

Q286. Answer: C

Explanation: Any breach threatens sterility. Placing in sterile over-bag and notifying lab allows evaluation and traceability. Using or discarding without documentation violates chain-of-custody and endangers recipient safety.
SubChapter: Product Integrity Control

Q287. Answer: A

Explanation: Radiation damages oral mucosa; bland saline or sodium-bicarbonate rinses prevent infection and promote healing. Salt or acidic agents worsen irritation; hard food increases trauma. Education enhances compliance with oral care protocols.
SubChapter: Conditioning Mucositis Care

Q288. Answer: A

Explanation: Hypertension with dizziness may indicate DMSO toxicity. Stopping infusion prevents cardiovascular strain and allows evaluation. Continuing even slowly may escalate symptoms. Antacids do not treat vascular effects.
SubChapter: Cryoprotectant Toxicity

Q289. Answer: A

Explanation: Mechanical obstruction is common; inspecting tubing and position corrects flow safely. Adjusting anticoagulant or restarting before assessment risks error and delays. Stopping procedure wastes time and resources unnecessarily.
SubChapter: Apheresis Troubleshooting

Q290. Answer: D

Explanation: Fever following infusion may indicate contamination or reaction; immediate cessation and assessment prevent deterioration. Simply medicating or waiting risks sepsis. Prompt provider notification ensures cultures and therapy.
SubChapter: Post-Infusion Reaction

Q291. Answer: A

Explanation: Pain may indicate infection or malposition. Inspecting for redness, swelling, or drainage and cleansing reduces risk. Continuing without assessment may worsen injury. Heat can mask inflammation.
SubChapter: Access Site Care

Q292. Answer: A

Explanation: Electrolyte imbalances, especially hyponatremia, often cause altered mental status during conditioning due to fluid shifts or medications. Immediate correction prevents seizures. Blood counts or liver enzymes are less urgent for neurologic symptoms.
SubChapter: Conditioning Metabolic Monitoring

Q293. Answer: A

Explanation: Garlic odor arises from DMSO vapor; harmless but unpleasant. Reassurance normalizes expectation. Stopping infusion is unnecessary; filtering or ventilation adjustments provide no clinical benefit.
SubChapter: Cryoprotectant Education

Q294. Answer: D

Explanation: Red urine may signal hemolysis from incompatibility or product damage. Immediate cessation and evaluation avert renal injury. Reassurance or fluids alone delay management. Continuing exposes patient to worsening reaction.
SubChapter: Compatibility Reaction Response

Q295. Answer: A

Explanation: Lightheadedness likely due to mild vasovagal response. Trendelenburg position restores cerebral perfusion. Coffee or arm-raising ineffective; stopping device may not be needed once symptoms resolve.

SubChapter: Donor Safety – Vasovagal Care

Q296. Answer: A

Explanation: Precise 37 °C ensures rapid, uniform thaw preserving cell viability. Lower temperatures allow ice damage; higher cause heat injury. Strict temperature control safeguards engraftment success.

SubChapter: Thawing Technique Quality

Q297. Answer: A

Explanation: Respiratory distress could indicate pulmonary reaction or embolic event; assessing oxygen saturation and alerting provider ensures prompt intervention. Continuing infusion endangers airway stability. Symptomatic cough relief is secondary.

SubChapter: Infusion Complications – Respiratory

Q298. Answer: C

Explanation: Blood exposure to extracorporeal circuit lowers body temperature; warming improves comfort without altering collection. Stopping or increasing rate affects yield; diuretics irrelevant.

SubChapter: Donor Comfort Measures

Q299. Answer: A

Explanation: Mesna binds acrolein to neutralize urotoxicity; prompt use prevents hemorrhagic cystitis progression. Analgesics or dietary changes offer no protection. Antibiotics address infection, not chemical injury.

SubChapter: Conditioning Uroprotection

Q300. Answer: A

Explanation: Maintaining sterility is crucial; replacing the set prevents contamination. Rapid reconnection or taping breaches asepsis and risks infection. Safe handling avoids product waste and sepsis.

SubChapter: Infusion Sterility Management

Questions (301-400)

Q301. Donor experiences headache after G-CSF. What should nurse teach?

A. Mild and temporary

B. Sign of infection

C. Need for steroids

D. Stop drug now

Q302. Patient post-infusion reports fever within 4 hours. Nurse should first:

A. Ignore mild rise

B. Give antipyretic

C. Observe longer

D. Assess and culture

Q303. During infusion, patient suddenly feels warmth and facial flushing. What is nurse's first action?

A. Stop infusion now

B. Slow rate slightly

C. Give fluids fast

D. Reassure calmly

Q304. Apheresis machine alarms "air detected." What should the nurse do first?

A. Clamp line fast

B. Continue slow

C. Check clamps

D. Silence alarm

Q305. Patient reports chest tightness during thawed-cell infusion. What is the next nursing step?

A. Stop infusion

B. Slow rate

C. Recheck ID

D. Offer water

Q306. Donor complains of hand cramps while collecting cells. What should nurse provide?

A. Extra fluids

B. Candy snack

C. IV calcium

D. Warm blanket

Q307. Patient becomes hypotensive near end of infusion. Which action is priority?

A. Stop infusion

B. Give fluids

C. Raise legs

D. Call provider

Q308. A patient 10 days post–allogeneic transplant develops fever and neutropenia. Which intervention should be initiated first?

A. Broad-spectrum antibiotics

B. Blood cultures only

C. Antifungal therapy immediately

D. Delay until ANC >500

Q309. Which immunosuppressive drug is most commonly used to prevent acute GVHD?

A. Cyclophosphamide

B. Tacrolimus

C. Rituximab

D. Methotrexate

Q310. The first sign of engraftment after hematopoietic stem cell transplantation is typically:
A. Rising hemoglobin
B. Increase in platelet count
C. Absolute neutrophil count >500 for 3 days
D. Decrease in infection rate
Q311. Which organism is most commonly associated with pneumonia in the early post-transplant period (day 0–30)?
A. Aspergillus species
B. Pneumocystis jirovecii
C. Cytomegalovirus (CMV)
D. Gram-negative bacteria
Q312. A patient on cyclosporine presents with tremor and hypertension. What is the most likely cause?
A. Drug toxicity
B. Infection
C. GVHD flare
D. Electrolyte imbalance
Q313. Which condition results from donor T-cell activation against host tissues within the first 100 days post-transplant?
A. Chronic GVHD
B. Acute GVHD
C. Graft rejection
D. Engraftment syndrome
Q314. Cytokine Release Syndrome (CRS) is most commonly associated with which therapy?
A. Autologous transplant
B. Radiation therapy
C. CAR-T cell therapy
D. Antifungal therapy
Q315. Which intervention best prevents veno-occlusive disease (VOD)?
A. Early steroid therapy
B. Ursodiol administration
C. Ganciclovir prophylaxis
D. Platelet transfusion support
Q316. During neutropenia, which dietary approach minimizes infection risk?
A. High-protein diet
B. Neutropenic (low microbial) diet
C. Gluten-free diet
D. High-calorie diet
Q317. What electrolyte imbalance is commonly caused by tacrolimus?
A. Hyperkalemia
B. Hypocalcemia
C. Hyponatremia
D. Hypokalemia
Q318. Which condition presents with fever, rash, and pulmonary infiltrates during neutrophil recovery?
A. Engraftment syndrome
B. Sepsis
C. Chronic GVHD

D. CMV reactivation
Q319. Which of the following is a hallmark feature of acute GVHD of the liver?
A. Elevated alkaline phosphatase and bilirubin
B. Neutropenia
C. Elevated creatinine
D. Hypocalcemia
Q320. A day +15 transplant patient has diarrhea exceeding 1 liter/day. Which diagnostic test is most appropriate?
A. Stool guaiac
B. Colon biopsy
C. Abdominal ultrasound
D. Plain abdominal X-ray
Q321. Which antimicrobial prophylaxis is essential for Pneumocystis jirovecii prevention?
A. Trimethoprim-sulfamethoxazole
B. Levofloxacin
C. Voriconazole
D. Acyclovir
Q322. Which symptom most strongly suggests sepsis in a neutropenic transplant patient?
A. High fever with rigors
B. Dry cough
C. Rash
D. Mild fatigue
Q323. What is the most common cause of death during the first 30 days post-transplant?
A. Relapse of malignancy
B. Sepsis
C. Chronic GVHD
D. Organ failure
Q324. What finding distinguishes engraftment syndrome from infection?
A. Elevated procalcitonin
B. Negative cultures
C. Neutropenia
D. Hypoxia
Q325. Which therapy prevents cytomegalovirus (CMV) reactivation in high-risk recipients?
A. Acyclovir
B. Levofloxacin
C. Amphotericin B
D. Ganciclovir or valganciclovir
Q326. Which blood product modification minimizes GVHD risk in transfused transplant recipients?
A. Leukoreduction
B. Irradiation
C. Washing
D. Cryopreservation
Q327. What primary nursing education is vital for patients discharged early post-transplant?
A. Resume normal diet
B. Avoid crowds and monitor temperature
C. Discontinue prophylactic antimicrobials
D. Limit fluid intake
Q328. Which finding indicates successful platelet engraftment after transplantation?

A. Platelet count >20,000/μL for three days without transfusion
B. Absence of petechiae
C. Hemoglobin stability
D. Resolution of fever

Q329. A patient on tacrolimus has rising creatinine levels. What is the most appropriate nursing action?
A. Hold the dose and notify the provider
B. Administer IV fluids
C. Continue medication and recheck later
D. Give potassium supplements

Q330. What is the primary goal of immunosuppressive therapy in early post-transplant care?
A. Prevent infection
B. Reduce cytokine production
C. Prevent graft rejection and GVHD
D. Stimulate engraftment

Q331. What symptom is most specific for gastrointestinal GVHD?
A. Jaundice
B. Diarrhea with abdominal pain
C. Mucositis
D. Fever

Q332. Which antifungal is preferred for prophylaxis during neutropenia?
A. Amphotericin B
B. Fluconazole
C. Caspofungin
D. Itraconazole

Q333. Which lab trend suggests successful engraftment?
A. Stable hematocrit
B. Progressive increase in ANC, platelets, and reticulocytes
C. Decreasing bilirubin
D. Stable creatinine

Q334. Which nursing intervention reduces risk of infection in a neutropenic patient?
A. Use of fresh flowers in the room
B. Encouraging visitors
C. Strict hand hygiene
D. Removing face mask indoors

Q335. The best indicator for early detection of sepsis in post-transplant patients is:
A. Drop in platelet count
B. New-onset fever
C. Weight loss
D. Tachycardia alone

Q336. What is the key factor contributing to acute GVHD severity?
A. Donor-recipient HLA disparity
B. Age of the patient
C. Use of growth factors
D. Blood type mismatch

Q337. What is the first-line therapy for acute GVHD of the skin?
A. Methotrexate
B. Systemic corticosteroids

C. Tacrolimus alone
D. Antithymocyte globulin

Q338. A patient with fever and hypotension on day +7 post-transplant is at greatest risk for:
A. Fungal sepsis
B. Bacterial sepsis
C. Viral reactivation
D. Acute GVHD

Q339. Which nutritional goal supports mucosal healing after conditioning therapy?
A. High-fat intake
B. Increased protein and calorie support
C. Low-fiber diet only
D. Vitamin supplementation alone

Q340. What is the primary cause of engraftment failure?
A. Infection
B. Immunosuppression overdose
C. GVHD
D. HLA mismatch or inadequate stem cell dose

Q341. A transplant patient develops dyspnea, weight gain, and hepatomegaly by day +18. What condition is suspected?
A. Acute GVHD
B. Veno-occlusive disease
C. Sepsis
D. Engraftment syndrome

Q342. What intervention is critical for preventing bacterial infections during neutropenia?
A. Oral ciprofloxacin prophylaxis
B. Antiviral prophylaxis
C. Low-sodium diet
D. Iron supplementation

Q343. Which early symptom suggests pulmonary toxicity from conditioning therapy?
A. Cough and dyspnea
B. Diarrhea
C. Jaundice
D. Weight gain

Q344. Which patient education topic is most important before discharge on immunosuppressive therapy?
A. Avoid abrupt discontinuation
B. Take medication with grapefruit juice
C. Skip doses when nauseated
D. Stop therapy after 2 weeks

Q345. Which laboratory marker indicates early sepsis progression?
A. Elevated procalcitonin
B. Decreased hematocrit
C. High albumin
D. Low bilirubin

Q346. Which infection is best prevented through vaccination after immune recovery?
A. CMV
B. Streptococcus pneumoniae
C. Aspergillus fumigatus

D. HSV

Q347. Which electrolyte imbalance signals early tumor lysis or cytokine release post-engraftment?

A. Hyperkalemia
B. Hypomagnesemia
C. Hypernatremia
D. Hypocalcemia

Q348. What is the most likely cause of persistent fever in a patient with neutropenia unresponsive to antibiotics?

A. Fungal infection
B. Viral infection
C. Bacterial resistance
D. GVHD

Q349. Which sign differentiates veno-occlusive disease (VOD) from fluid overload?

A. Weight gain
B. Painful hepatomegaly
C. Peripheral edema
D. Elevated BNP

Q350. The most appropriate management for early signs of engraftment syndrome includes:

A. Broad-spectrum antibiotics
B. High-dose corticosteroids
C. Antifungal prophylaxis
D. Reduction of immunosuppressants

Q351. Which prophylaxis is used to prevent CMV reactivation in seropositive transplant recipients?

A. Levofloxacin
B. Ganciclovir
C. Acyclovir
D. Fluconazole

Q352. Which condition is characterized by rising bilirubin, hepatomegaly, and ascites within 20 days post-transplant?

A. Acute GVHD
B. Veno-occlusive disease
C. Engraftment syndrome
D. Sepsis

Q353. A patient with severe neutropenia develops cough and pleuritic pain. What diagnostic test is most useful?

A. Sputum culture
B. Blood culture
C. Chest X-ray
D. High-resolution chest CT

Q354. What intervention reduces severity of cytokine release syndrome after CAR-T therapy?

A. Tocilizumab administration
B. Steroid discontinuation
C. Fluid restriction
D. Granulocyte transfusion

Q355. Which clinical sign differentiates acute GVHD from engraftment syndrome?

A. Rash
B. Diarrhea
C. Timing after transplant

D. Fever

Q356. What immediate step should be taken for a post-transplant patient with fever >38.3°C and ANC <500?

A. Notify physician and start empiric antibiotics
B. Wait for culture results
C. Begin antivirals
D. Administer diuretics

Q357. Which laboratory trend supports diagnosis of engraftment?

A. Stable creatinine and bilirubin
B. Increasing ANC and platelet counts
C. Decreasing lactate
D. Falling hemoglobin

Q358. What is the most appropriate management for grade III acute GVHD involving the GI tract?

A. Topical corticosteroids only
B. High-dose systemic corticosteroids
C. Reduction in tacrolimus dose
D. Observation and hydration

Q359. Which prophylaxis prevents reactivation of herpes simplex virus post-transplant?

A. Acyclovir
B. Ganciclovir
C. Levofloxacin
D. Fluconazole

Q360. Which early post-transplant complication is characterized by fever, rash, and pulmonary infiltrates without infection?

A. Engraftment syndrome
B. Acute GVHD
C. Sepsis
D. CMV pneumonia

Q361. What is the recommended duration for antimicrobial prophylaxis after allogeneic transplant?

A. Until ANC >500 and mucositis resolves
B. One week post-discharge
C. Two months regardless of counts
D. When antibiotics finish inpatient

Q362. What is the preferred management for acute GVHD unresponsive to steroids?

A. Increase tacrolimus dose
B. Add ruxolitinib or extracorporeal photopheresis
C. Discontinue immunosuppression
D. Switch to methotrexate

Q363. What major cause of death occurs during the early post-transplant period besides infection?

A. Multi-organ failure from conditioning toxicity
B. Chronic GVHD
C. Disease relapse
D. Late cardiac toxicity

Q364. Which nutritional modification helps patients with severe mucositis after conditioning therapy?

A. Parenteral nutrition
B. High-fiber diet
C. Spicy food for appetite
D. Fluid restriction

Q365. Which factor increases risk for severe GVHD?
A. Younger recipient
B. Peripheral blood stem cell graft source
C. HLA-matched sibling donor
D. Reduced-intensity conditioning
Q366. What nursing priority applies to a patient with new-onset dyspnea after transplant?
A. Evaluate for pulmonary infection and VOD
B. Encourage deep breathing only
C. Reduce fluids and observe
D. Start diuretics
Q367. What should caregivers monitor daily for patients discharged after transplant?
A. Temperature and signs of infection
B. Urine output only
C. Weight gain
D. Blood pressure twice weekly
Q368. A patient develops elevated bilirubin and right upper quadrant pain on day +12 post-transplant. What is the most likely cause?
A. Sepsis
B. Veno-occlusive disease
C. GVHD of the liver
D. Drug-induced liver injury
Q369. Which medication combination is most often used for GVHD prophylaxis?
A. Tacrolimus and methotrexate
B. Prednisone and rituximab
C. Cyclosporine and azathioprine
D. Sirolimus and ganciclovir
Q370. A neutropenic patient develops oral ulcers with pseudomembranes. Which organism is the most probable cause?
A. Candida albicans
B. Herpes simplex virus
C. Cytomegalovirus
D. Streptococcus pneumoniae
Q371. What laboratory finding confirms neutrophil engraftment?
A. ANC >500/mm^3 for three consecutive days
B. Hemoglobin rise of 2 g/dL
C. Platelet count >100,000/µL
D. Decrease in C-reactive protein
Q372. Which symptom warrants immediate investigation for acute GI GVHD?
A. Weight gain
B. Abdominal pain and persistent diarrhea
C. Oral mucositis
D. Constipation
Q373. What is the most common infection source during the first two weeks post-transplant?
A. Endogenous bacterial flora
B. Community-acquired viruses
C. Airborne fungi
D. Reactivated CMV
Q374. Which immunosuppressive drug requires close monitoring for nephrotoxicity?

A. Tacrolimus
B. Methotrexate
C. Prednisone
D. Sirolimus

Q375. A patient experiences fever, rash, and pulmonary infiltrates on day +10. Cultures are negative. Which condition is likely?
A. Engraftment syndrome
B. Bacterial pneumonia
C. Acute GVHD
D. CMV pneumonitis

Q376. Which intervention is most important to prevent bacterial translocation in severe mucositis?
A. Maintain oral hygiene with saline rinses
B. Use chlorhexidine mouthwash only
C. Limit oral fluids
D. Delay mouth care until healing

Q377. What is the preferred treatment for steroid-refractory acute GVHD?
A. Cyclosporine alone
B. Cyclophosphamide
C. Methotrexate
D. Ruxolitinib

Q378. Which electrolyte imbalance is commonly associated with cyclosporine therapy?
A. Hyperkalemia and hypomagnesemia
B. Hyponatremia
C. Hypokalemia
D. Hypercalcemia

Q379. What is the most effective measure to prevent Pneumocystis jirovecii infection post-transplant?
A. Trimethoprim-sulfamethoxazole
B. Ciprofloxacin
C. Amphotericin B
D. Fluconazole

Q380. A patient with suspected GVHD undergoes liver biopsy. Which finding supports the diagnosis?
A. Bile duct damage and lymphocytic infiltration
B. Fatty degeneration
C. Necrosis without inflammation
D. Iron overload

Q381. What infection commonly occurs after engraftment but before full immune recovery?
A. Influenza
B. Bacterial sepsis
C. Candida fungemia
D. CMV reactivation

Q382. What nursing action is critical during tocilizumab administration for cytokine release syndrome?
A. Monitor for hypotension and oxygen saturation changes
B. Restrict IV fluids
C. Increase tacrolimus dose
D. Avoid corticosteroids

Q383. Which patient is at highest risk for delayed engraftment?

A. Recipient of cord blood transplant
B. HLA-matched sibling transplant
C. Autologous transplant
D. Haploidentical donor

Q384. What education is essential for caregivers regarding infection prevention at home?
A. Maintain strict hand hygiene and avoid sick contacts
B. Allow pets in the patient's room
C. Avoid all fruits and vegetables
D. Use only bottled water for drinking

Q385. What is the primary reason for using irradiated blood products post-transplant?
A. Prevent bacterial contamination
B. Reduce iron overload
C. Prevent transfusion-associated GVHD
D. Prolong shelf life

Q386. Which prophylaxis helps prevent fungal pneumonia during prolonged neutropenia?
A. Posaconazole
B. Acyclovir
C. Ciprofloxacin
D. Ganciclovir

Q387. What complication does early immune reconstitution increase risk for in mismatched transplants?
A. Cytokine release syndrome
B. Chronic GVHD
C. Tumor lysis syndrome
D. Iron overload

Q388. A patient presents with jaundice, diarrhea, and a maculopapular rash on day +35 post-transplant. What is the most likely diagnosis?
A. CMV infection
B. Chronic GVHD
C. Engraftment syndrome
D. Acute GVHD

Q389. Which patient is at highest risk of CMV reactivation after transplant?
A. Seropositive recipient with seronegative donor
B. Seronegative recipient with seronegative donor
C. Autologous transplant patient
D. Cord blood recipient

Q390. What is the most common cause of noninfectious fever during engraftment?
A. Cytokine release
B. Transfusion reaction
C. Drug hypersensitivity
D. Organ rejection

Q391. Which intervention reduces risk of sepsis in a neutropenic patient with mucositis?
A. Aggressive oral care and saline rinses
B. Broad antifungal prophylaxis only
C. Reduction of antibiotic use
D. Allowing raw fruits and vegetables

Q392. Which organ is most frequently affected by early veno-occlusive disease?
A. Heart

B. Lungs
C. Kidneys
D. Liver

Q393. What lab result suggests early CMV reactivation?
A. Positive CMV PCR
B. Elevated alkaline phosphatase
C. Decreased white blood cell count
D. Positive blood culture

Q394. Which dietary instruction is most appropriate for neutropenic patients?
A. Avoid raw or undercooked foods
B. Increase dairy intake
C. Restrict carbohydrates
D. Limit protein sources

Q395. Which finding supports diagnosis of engraftment syndrome?
A. Fever, rash, and pulmonary infiltrates without infection
B. Hypotension and jaundice
C. Neutropenia with diarrhea
D. Positive bacterial cultures

Q396. Which prophylactic agent prevents HSV reactivation post-transplant?
A. Trimethoprim-sulfamethoxazole
B. Ciprofloxacin
C. Amphotericin B
D. Acyclovir

Q397. What early symptom distinguishes sepsis from cytokine release syndrome?
A. Positive blood cultures
B. Fever
C. Rash
D. Hypotension

Q398. Which diagnostic test is most specific for confirming acute GVHD?
A. Biopsy of affected tissue
B. CBC with differential
C. Serum bilirubin measurement
D. Stool cultures

Q399. What preventive strategy reduces the risk of fungal infections in high-risk allogeneic transplant recipients?
A. HEPA filtration rooms
B. Vitamin supplementation
C. Oral probiotics
D. Zinc therapy

Q400. What electrolyte imbalance can occur with amphotericin B therapy?
A. Hyperkalemia
B. Hypernatremia
C. Hypocalcemia
D. Hypokalemia and hypomagnesemia

Answer key and Explanation (301-400)

Q301. Answer: A

Explanation: Headache and bone pain are common transient effects from marrow stimulation. Analgesics relieve discomfort. Stopping G-CSF jeopardizes adequate mobilization. Steroids unnecessary unless severe inflammation occurs.

SubChapter: Donor Education – G-CSF Effects

Q302. Answer: D

Explanation: Early fever may indicate contaminated product or reaction. Immediate assessment, vital monitoring, and cultures prevent septic progression. Antipyretics before evaluation obscure findings. Prompt action aligns with transplant infection-control protocols.

SubChapter: Post-Infusion Monitoring

Q303. Answer: A

Explanation: Flushing and warmth may indicate allergic or DMSO-related reaction. Stopping infusion halts exposure and allows assessment before further deterioration. Slowing rate or reassurance alone delays life-saving interventions. Rapid fluids without evaluation risk worsening hemodynamic instability.

SubChapter: Infusion Reaction – Initial Response

Q304. Answer: A

Explanation: Air entry can cause embolism. Immediate clamping prevents further air introduction, followed by air removal and line inspection. Continuing or muting alarm jeopardizes donor safety. Verification ensures system integrity before restarting the circuit.

SubChapter: Collection Safety – Air Management

Q305. Answer: A

Explanation: Chest pressure during infusion suggests hypersensitivity or DMSO toxicity. Stopping infusion allows rapid assessment and intervention with antihistamines or corticosteroids if indicated. Continuing even slowly risks progression to severe cardiopulmonary compromise.

SubChapter: Infusion Reaction – Cardiopulmonary

Q306. Answer: C

Explanation: Citrate binds ionized calcium, producing muscle cramps and paresthesias. IV calcium corrects imbalance quickly and prevents tetany. Snacks or warmth may comfort but do not resolve metabolic cause; fluid bolus alone is ineffective.

SubChapter: Collection – Citrate Toxicity Relief

Q307. Answer: A

Explanation: Stopping infusion immediately prevents additional exposure to potential causative agent such as reaction or contamination. Subsequent management includes fluids and positioning after stabilization. Acting sequentially safeguards airway, circulation, and product traceability.

SubChapter: Infusion Reaction – Hypotension Response

Q308. Answer: A

Explanation: Febrile neutropenia in early post-transplant demands prompt empiric broad-spectrum antibiotic initiation to prevent sepsis. Option B delays care; Option C is premature without bacterial coverage; Option D risks progression to septic shock. Early broad-spectrum therapy reduces mortality by covering gram-negative and gram-positive organisms.

SubChapter: Infection Prevention and Management

Q309. Answer: B

Explanation: Tacrolimus, a calcineurin inhibitor, is the cornerstone for acute GVHD prophylaxis, often combined with methotrexate. Cyclophosphamide is used post-transplant for GVHD prevention but not as first-line maintenance; Rituximab targets B-cells for specific diseases. Tacrolimus maintains T-cell suppression during early immune reconstitution to prevent donor T-cell activation.

SubChapter: Immunosuppressive Therapy

Q310. Answer: C
Explanation: Engraftment is defined by achieving an ANC >500/mm^3 for three consecutive days, indicating marrow recovery. Platelets and hemoglobin normalize later. Infection rates decline only after stable immune reconstitution. This metric signifies successful neutrophil production from donor cells.
SubChapter: Hematologic and Immune Reconstitution
Q311. Answer: D
Explanation: Early post-transplant infections are primarily bacterial, especially gram-negative pathogens like Pseudomonas and E. coli, due to neutropenia and mucosal injury. Aspergillus and CMV dominate later phases. Prompt empiric antibiotic therapy is vital to prevent sepsis-related mortality during this neutropenic period.
SubChapter: Infection Prevention and Management
Q312. Answer: A
Explanation: Cyclosporine toxicity manifests as tremor, hypertension, and nephrotoxicity due to calcineurin inhibition affecting renal perfusion. Infection and GVHD flare show different systemic symptoms. Monitoring drug levels prevents renal and neurotoxic complications during immunosuppressive therapy.
SubChapter: Immunosuppressive Therapy
Q313. Answer: B
Explanation: Acute GVHD arises within the first 100 days due to donor T-cell–mediated immune attack on recipient tissues, primarily skin, liver, and GI tract. Chronic GVHD develops later; graft rejection involves host immunity, and engraftment syndrome reflects cytokine release during marrow recovery.
SubChapter: Acute GVHD
Q314. Answer: C
Explanation: CRS results from immune activation following CAR-T or donor lymphocyte infusions, leading to systemic inflammation with fever, hypotension, and hypoxia. Autologous and radiation therapies do not typically trigger CRS. Early recognition and IL-6 blockade (e.g., tocilizumab) are critical for management.
SubChapter: Immune Reconstitution
Q315. Answer: B
Explanation: Ursodiol reduces hepatic injury by stabilizing bile flow and decreasing endothelial activation, preventing VOD after conditioning regimens. Steroids do not prevent VOD; ganciclovir targets viral infections, not hepatic injury. Platelet transfusion treats thrombocytopenia but does not influence VOD pathogenesis.
SubChapter: Acute System-Specific Complications
Q316. Answer: B
Explanation: A neutropenic diet restricts raw produce, unpasteurized foods, and undercooked meats to reduce microbial exposure during immunosuppression. This approach decreases bacterial translocation risk in patients with mucositis and neutropenia. High-protein or calorie diets do not specifically prevent infections.
SubChapter: Nutritional Support
Q317. Answer: A
Explanation: Tacrolimus induces hyperkalemia and nephrotoxicity through renal tubular dysfunction and reduced potassium excretion. Monitoring renal function and serum potassium is essential. Hyponatremia and hypocalcemia are less characteristic, and hypokalemia occurs more with diuretic use than immunosuppression.
SubChapter: Immunosuppressive Therapy
Q318. Answer: A

Explanation: Engraftment syndrome is a cytokine-driven inflammatory process occurring during neutrophil recovery, presenting with fever, rash, and noninfectious pulmonary infiltrates. It differs from sepsis (infectious), GVHD (immune attack on tissues), and CMV (viral reactivation). Corticosteroids often resolve symptoms promptly.
SubChapter: Immune Reconstitution

Q319. Answer: A

Explanation: Liver GVHD presents with cholestatic enzyme elevations—alkaline phosphatase and bilirubin—reflecting bile duct injury from donor T-cell infiltration. Creatinine changes indicate renal injury, not hepatic GVHD. Neutropenia and hypocalcemia are unrelated systemic findings.
SubChapter: Acute GVHD

Q320. Answer: B

Explanation: Persistent watery diarrhea post-transplant necessitates colon biopsy to differentiate acute GI GVHD from infectious etiologies. Histologic confirmation identifies crypt apoptosis and mucosal inflammation. Stool tests detect infection but cannot confirm GVHD; imaging adds little diagnostic value.
SubChapter: Acute GVHD

Q321. Answer: A

Explanation: Trimethoprim-sulfamethoxazole is the gold-standard prophylactic for Pneumocystis jirovecii pneumonia post-transplant. Fluoroquinolones target bacteria, voriconazole covers fungi, and acyclovir covers herpesviruses. Without TMP-SMX, risk of life-threatening opportunistic pneumonia significantly increases.
SubChapter: Infection Prevention and Management

Q322. Answer: A

Explanation: Fever with chills or rigors in neutropenia signals possible sepsis, warranting immediate cultures and empiric antibiotic therapy. Other symptoms like cough or rash may indicate localized infections but not systemic bacteremia. Delay in treatment dramatically increases mortality.
SubChapter: Sepsis Management

Q323. Answer: B

Explanation: Sepsis dominates early post-transplant mortality due to profound neutropenia and mucosal barrier disruption. Chronic GVHD and relapse occur later; organ failure typically follows severe infection. Vigilant monitoring and early empiric antibiotics improve survival during this vulnerable phase.
SubChapter: Sepsis Management

Q324. Answer: B

Explanation: Engraftment syndrome mimics infection but shows negative cultures, supporting an inflammatory rather than microbial etiology. Fever and pulmonary infiltrates occur in both, but culture negativity alongside neutrophil recovery helps differentiate it from bacterial sepsis.
SubChapter: Immune Reconstitution

Q325. Answer: D

Explanation: Ganciclovir or its oral analogue valganciclovir provides effective CMV prophylaxis for seropositive recipients or donor-recipient mismatches. Acyclovir lacks CMV activity; amphotericin targets fungi, and levofloxacin prevents bacterial infections, not viral.
SubChapter: Infection Prevention and Management

Q326. Answer: B

Explanation: Irradiation inactivates donor lymphocytes, preventing transfusion-associated GVHD in immunocompromised recipients. Leukoreduction reduces febrile reactions but not GVHD. Washing removes plasma proteins for allergic reactions; cryopreservation applies to stem cell storage.
SubChapter: Hematologic and Transfusion Support

Q327. Answer: B

Explanation: Early discharge education emphasizes strict infection control—avoiding crowds, hand hygiene, and daily temperature monitoring—to detect sepsis early. Continuing prophylactic antimicrobials and adequate hydration are also crucial. Returning to normal diet or reducing fluids risks infection and dehydration.
SubChapter: Patient and Caregiver Education

Q328. Answer: A

Explanation: Platelet engraftment is achieved when counts exceed 20,000/µL for at least three consecutive days without transfusion support. This milestone signifies marrow recovery and functional thrombopoiesis. Other findings, like fever resolution or hemoglobin stability, may occur independently of platelet recovery.
SubChapter: Hematologic and Immune Reconstitution

Q329. Answer: A

Explanation: Tacrolimus nephrotoxicity manifests as rising serum creatinine. Immediate notification and holding the dose prevent progression to renal failure. Hydration may help, but dose evaluation is essential. Potassium supplementation can worsen hyperkalemia associated with tacrolimus use.
SubChapter: Immunosuppressive Therapy

Q330. Answer: C

Explanation: Immunosuppressive therapy prevents graft-versus-host and graft rejection reactions by inhibiting T-cell activation. While infection prevention and cytokine control are secondary benefits, the main therapeutic aim is to maintain immune tolerance between donor and recipient tissues.
SubChapter: Immunosuppressive Therapy

Q331. Answer: B

Explanation: Acute GI GVHD typically presents as profuse watery diarrhea with cramping due to immune-mediated mucosal injury. Jaundice indicates hepatic involvement, mucositis occurs from conditioning toxicity, and fever is nonspecific. Colonoscopy and biopsy confirm the diagnosis.
SubChapter: Acute GVHD

Q332. Answer: B

Explanation: Fluconazole is the standard antifungal prophylaxis during early neutropenia, effectively preventing Candida infections with minimal toxicity. Amphotericin B causes nephrotoxicity, and echinocandins or itraconazole are reserved for broader or resistant fungal coverage.
SubChapter: Infection Prevention and Management

Q333. Answer: B

Explanation: Simultaneous rises in neutrophil, platelet, and reticulocyte counts indicate multi-lineage marrow recovery. This trend confirms effective engraftment and hematopoietic restoration. Other lab values may reflect organ function but not marrow activity.
SubChapter: Hematologic and Immune Reconstitution

Q334. Answer: C

Explanation: Meticulous hand hygiene remains the most effective infection control measure in neutropenic patients. Flowers and frequent visitors increase exposure risk. Masks protect against airborne pathogens and should be used during early recovery phases.
SubChapter: Infection Prevention and Management

Q335. Answer: B

Explanation: Fever is the most sensitive and early indicator of sepsis in immunocompromised patients. It warrants immediate investigation and antibiotic initiation. Other symptoms like tachycardia or thrombocytopenia appear later in disease progression.
SubChapter: Sepsis Management

Q336. Answer: A

Explanation: HLA mismatch triggers donor T-cell activation against host antigens, leading to more severe GVHD. Age and growth factors influence tolerance and recovery but are less predictive. ABO mismatches rarely cause significant GVHD.
SubChapter: Acute GVHD

Q337. Answer: B
Explanation: Systemic corticosteroids remain the first-line treatment for acute GVHD, reducing T-cell proliferation and inflammation. Tacrolimus continues as baseline prophylaxis but does not reverse established GVHD. Antithymocyte globulin is reserved for steroid-refractory cases.
SubChapter: Acute GVHD

Q338. Answer: B
Explanation: Early post-transplant sepsis, particularly in the neutropenic phase, is usually bacterial, originating from gram-negative flora. Fungal and viral infections occur later when immunosuppression persists. Rapid empiric antibacterial coverage is life-saving at this stage.
SubChapter: Sepsis Management

Q339. Answer: B
Explanation: Adequate protein and caloric intake promote mucosal repair, immune recovery, and overall metabolic balance after conditioning injury. Restrictive or supplement-only diets cannot meet these recovery demands, and high fat may worsen gastrointestinal distress.
SubChapter: Nutritional Support

Q340. Answer: D
Explanation: Engraftment failure most often results from insufficient viable stem cell infusion or donor-recipient HLA disparity causing graft rejection. Infection and GVHD can complicate engraftment but are secondary contributors. Dose adequacy and immune compatibility are critical for success.
SubChapter: Hematologic and Immune Reconstitution

Q341. Answer: B
Explanation: Veno-occlusive disease presents with hepatomegaly, ascites, weight gain, and right upper quadrant pain due to hepatic venous obstruction after conditioning regimens. Engraftment syndrome involves fever and rash; GVHD affects skin and GI tract.
SubChapter: Acute System-Specific Complications

Q342. Answer: A
Explanation: Fluoroquinolone prophylaxis, such as ciprofloxacin, reduces gram-negative bacterial infections during profound neutropenia. Antivirals and diet modifications have different indications, and iron supplementation offers no infection prevention benefit.
SubChapter: Infection Prevention and Management

Q343. Answer: A
Explanation: Cough and dyspnea in early post-transplant may indicate pulmonary toxicity from conditioning regimens, such as busulfan or radiation. Prompt evaluation prevents progression to interstitial pneumonitis. Other symptoms relate to hepatic or gastrointestinal systems.
SubChapter: Acute System-Specific Complications

Q344. Answer: A
Explanation: Abrupt cessation of immunosuppressants can precipitate acute GVHD or graft rejection. Patients must maintain strict adherence and consult clinicians before any dose change. Grapefruit juice increases drug levels, and skipping doses compromises immune stability.
SubChapter: Patient and Caregiver Education

Q345. Answer: A
Explanation: Elevated procalcitonin indicates bacterial infection and sepsis progression, even before culture confirmation. It helps guide antibiotic therapy escalation. Other lab values are less specific for systemic infection.

SubChapter: Sepsis Management

Q346. Answer: B

Explanation: Vaccination against encapsulated bacteria such as Streptococcus pneumoniae is essential after immune recovery to prevent post-transplant bacterial pneumonia. CMV and HSV require antiviral prophylaxis, and fungal infections need antifungal agents.

SubChapter: Infection Prevention and Management

Q347. Answer: A

Explanation: Hyperkalemia is a hallmark of tumor lysis and cytokine-driven cellular breakdown during engraftment. It reflects rapid cell turnover and can lead to cardiac arrhythmias if untreated. Monitoring and hydration are critical preventive strategies.

SubChapter: Immune Reconstitution

Q348. Answer: A

Explanation: In persistent febrile neutropenia unresponsive to broad-spectrum antibiotics, invasive fungal infection—commonly Aspergillus or Candida—is suspected. Empiric antifungal therapy is initiated promptly. Viral reactivation or GVHD are less common early causes of prolonged fever.

SubChapter: Infection Prevention and Management

Q349. Answer: B

Explanation: Painful hepatomegaly and right upper quadrant tenderness are distinctive for VOD, caused by hepatic sinusoidal obstruction. Weight gain and edema occur in both conditions, but hepatic pain and rising bilirubin confirm VOD diagnosis.

SubChapter: Acute System-Specific Complications

Q350. Answer: B

Explanation: Engraftment syndrome, an inflammatory response during neutrophil recovery, is treated with corticosteroids to suppress cytokine-mediated injury. Antibiotics are used only if infection is suspected. Reducing immunosuppressants may worsen inflammation and graft injury.

SubChapter: Immune Reconstitution

Q351. Answer: B

Explanation: Ganciclovir is the antiviral agent of choice for CMV prophylaxis in seropositive patients or high-risk mismatches. It prevents viral replication during immunosuppression. Acyclovir targets HSV/VZV, and fluconazole addresses fungal, not viral, infections.

SubChapter: Infection Prevention and Management

Q352. Answer: B

Explanation: Veno-occlusive disease occurs early after conditioning due to endothelial damage, causing hepatic congestion, elevated bilirubin, and fluid retention. Engraftment syndrome lacks hepatomegaly, and GVHD involves skin or GI tract inflammation.

SubChapter: Acute System-Specific Complications

Q353. Answer: D

Explanation: High-resolution chest CT best detects early invasive fungal infection, revealing nodular or halo signs before X-ray changes appear. Sputum and blood cultures have low yield in neutropenic patients with pulmonary infection.

SubChapter: Infection Prevention and Management

Q354. Answer: A

Explanation: Tocilizumab, an IL-6 receptor antagonist, mitigates cytokine release syndrome by dampening inflammatory cascades. Steroid discontinuation worsens symptoms, and fluid restriction or granulocyte transfusion offer no cytokine modulation.

SubChapter: Immune Reconstitution

Q355. Answer: C

Explanation: Timing distinguishes engraftment syndrome, which occurs during neutrophil recovery, from acute GVHD, which develops days to weeks later after donor T-cell activation. Both may present with rash and fever, requiring biopsy for definitive differentiation.
SubChapter: Acute GVHD
Q356. Answer: A
Explanation: Febrile neutropenia constitutes a medical emergency; immediate empiric broad-spectrum antibiotics are initiated before culture results. Delay increases mortality risk. Antivirals and diuretics are inappropriate unless specific indications exist.
SubChapter: Sepsis Management
Q357. Answer: B
Explanation: A consistent rise in neutrophil and platelet counts indicates successful engraftment and marrow recovery. Organ function markers may remain stable, but hematologic indices directly confirm donor cell proliferation.
SubChapter: Hematologic and Immune Reconstitution
Q358. Answer: B
Explanation: Grade III GVHD requires aggressive systemic corticosteroid therapy to control intestinal inflammation and prevent perforation. Topical treatment is insufficient for severe disease, and reducing immunosuppressants would exacerbate tissue injury.
SubChapter: Acute GVHD
Q359. Answer: A
Explanation: Acyclovir effectively prevents HSV and VZV reactivation during immunosuppression. Ganciclovir targets CMV, fluconazole covers fungal infections, and levofloxacin is antibacterial. Continuous prophylaxis is essential until immune recovery.
SubChapter: Infection Prevention and Management
Q360. Answer: A
Explanation: Engraftment syndrome manifests as fever, rash, and noninfectious pulmonary infiltrates due to cytokine surge during neutrophil recovery. Absence of pathogens on culture supports diagnosis. Acute GVHD develops later with organ-specific involvement.
SubChapter: Immune Reconstitution
Q361. Answer: A
Explanation: Antimicrobial prophylaxis continues until neutrophil recovery and mucosal integrity return, reducing infection risk. Fixed durations are unsafe due to variable immune recovery among patients. Clinical judgment guides discontinuation timing.
SubChapter: Infection Prevention and Management
Q362. Answer: B
Explanation: Steroid-refractory acute GVHD responds to advanced therapies such as ruxolitinib or extracorporeal photopheresis, which target cytokine signaling and T-cell activity. Increasing calcineurin inhibitors alone rarely achieves control.
SubChapter: Acute GVHD
Q363. Answer: A
Explanation: Conditioning-related organ toxicity, especially hepatic and pulmonary, can cause early mortality aside from infection. Chronic GVHD and relapse occur later, and cardiac effects emerge months after therapy.
SubChapter: Acute System-Specific Complications
Q364. Answer: A
Explanation: Parenteral nutrition provides essential nutrients while bypassing the inflamed mucosa during severe mucositis. High-fiber or spicy foods worsen irritation, and fluid restriction impairs recovery. Early nutritional support prevents catabolism and infection.

SubChapter: Nutritional Support

Q365. Answer: B

Explanation: Peripheral blood grafts carry higher T-cell content, increasing GVHD risk compared to bone marrow or cord blood. Younger recipients tolerate GVHD better, and matched sibling donors minimize risk. Reduced-intensity regimens further lower GVHD severity.

SubChapter: Acute GVHD

Q366. Answer: A

Explanation: Dyspnea post-transplant may indicate infection, pulmonary edema, or VOD-related hepatic congestion. Prompt diagnostic workup prevents progression to respiratory failure. Supportive measures alone delay essential interventions.

SubChapter: Acute System-Specific Complications

Q367. Answer: A

Explanation: Daily temperature monitoring ensures early infection detection in immunocompromised patients. Prompt reporting of fever allows rapid intervention, reducing sepsis mortality. Other parameters, though useful, are secondary to infection surveillance.

SubChapter: Patient and Caregiver Education

Q368. Answer: B

Explanation: Veno-occlusive disease occurs early after conditioning therapy from sinusoidal endothelial injury. Typical findings include painful hepatomegaly, elevated bilirubin, and ascites. Liver GVHD develops later, and drug-induced injury lacks ascites or hepatomegaly. Early recognition improves outcomes with defibrotide therapy.

SubChapter: Acute System-Specific Complications

Q369. Answer: A

Explanation: Tacrolimus plus methotrexate remains the standard GVHD prophylaxis in allogeneic transplantation. This combination effectively suppresses T-cell activation while minimizing organ toxicity. Prednisone and rituximab treat established immune disease, while sirolimus and ganciclovir serve specific or adjunctive roles, not first-line prophylaxis.

SubChapter: Immunosuppressive Therapy

Q370. Answer: A

Explanation: Candida albicans commonly causes pseudomembranous oral lesions during neutropenia due to mucosal barrier damage and antibiotic use. HSV causes vesicular ulcers, not plaques; CMV typically affects the GI tract. Early antifungal prophylaxis with fluconazole prevents systemic dissemination.

SubChapter: Infection Prevention and Management

Q371. Answer: A

Explanation: Neutrophil engraftment is officially defined by an absolute neutrophil count exceeding $500/mm^3$ for three consecutive days. This indicates successful hematopoietic recovery. Hemoglobin and platelet changes occur later, while inflammatory markers fluctuate independently of engraftment status.

SubChapter: Hematologic and Immune Reconstitution

Q372. Answer: B

Explanation: Acute GI GVHD often presents with profuse watery diarrhea and cramping from immune-mediated mucosal injury. These symptoms require prompt biopsy confirmation to differentiate from infection. Mucositis is a chemotherapy effect, and constipation is unrelated.

SubChapter: Acute GVHD

Q373. Answer: A

Explanation: Early post-transplant infections usually originate from the patient's own bacterial flora due to mucosal barrier disruption and neutropenia. Viral reactivation and fungal infections occur later when immunosuppression persists. Early empiric antibiotics target gram-negative flora.

SubChapter: Infection Prevention and Management

Q374. Answer: A

Explanation: Tacrolimus is associated with dose-dependent nephrotoxicity caused by renal vasoconstriction. Regular drug level and creatinine monitoring are essential to prevent irreversible kidney damage. Methotrexate and sirolimus have different toxicity profiles, while prednisone rarely affects renal function.

SubChapter: Immunosuppressive Therapy

Q375. Answer: A

Explanation: Engraftment syndrome results from cytokine release during marrow recovery, causing fever, rash, and sterile pulmonary infiltrates. Negative cultures and timing near neutrophil recovery confirm diagnosis. GVHD and CMV pneumonitis occur later and show tissue-specific pathology.

SubChapter: Immune Reconstitution

Q376. Answer: A

Explanation: Gentle saline rinses maintain mucosal integrity and reduce bacterial colonization, lowering sepsis risk from translocation. Chlorhexidine may irritate ulcers; fluid limitation or neglecting oral care worsens infection risk and discomfort.

SubChapter: Nutritional Support

Q377. Answer: D

Explanation: Ruxolitinib, a JAK1/2 inhibitor, is approved for steroid-refractory GVHD, targeting cytokine signaling pathways. It provides better control and survival outcomes. Cyclophosphamide is preventive post-transplant; methotrexate and cyclosporine are baseline prophylactic agents.

SubChapter: Acute GVHD

Q378. Answer: A

Explanation: Cyclosporine causes renal tubular dysfunction, resulting in hyperkalemia and hypomagnesemia. Regular electrolyte monitoring prevents arrhythmias and neurotoxicity. Sodium and calcium levels remain mostly unaffected by this calcineurin inhibitor.

SubChapter: Immunosuppressive Therapy

Q379. Answer: A

Explanation: Trimethoprim-sulfamethoxazole remains the gold standard for Pneumocystis jirovecii prophylaxis in immunocompromised patients. It prevents life-threatening pneumonia effectively compared to other antimicrobials. Fluconazole and amphotericin target fungi, not Pneumocystis.

SubChapter: Infection Prevention and Management

Q380. Answer: A

Explanation: Hepatic GVHD causes bile duct epithelial apoptosis and lymphocytic infiltration, leading to cholestatic liver enzyme elevation. Fatty degeneration or necrosis are nonspecific, and iron overload reflects transfusion-related hemosiderosis, not GVHD.

SubChapter: Acute GVHD

Q381. Answer: D

Explanation: CMV reactivation typically arises during intermediate recovery (30–100 days) when cellular immunity is incomplete. Bacterial infections dominate early neutropenia, while viral and fungal reactivations emerge later under immunosuppression.

SubChapter: Infection Prevention and Management

Q382. Answer: A

Explanation: Tocilizumab can cause rapid hemodynamic improvement but requires close monitoring for hypotension, hypoxia, and fever changes. Supportive care ensures safety during IL-6 blockade. Fluid restriction or immunosuppressant adjustments are unnecessary during infusion.

SubChapter: Immune Reconstitution

Q383. Answer: A

Explanation: Cord blood transplants have fewer stem cells and immature immune components, causing slower engraftment compared to bone marrow or peripheral blood sources. Haploidentical grafts recover faster with modern conditioning.
SubChapter: Hematologic and Immune Reconstitution

Q384. Answer: A

Explanation: Hand hygiene and avoidance of ill contacts are key to reducing post-discharge infection risk. Pets and contaminated food pose additional hazards, but total dietary restriction or exclusive bottled water use is unnecessary.
SubChapter: Patient and Caregiver Education

Q385. Answer: C

Explanation: Irradiation inactivates donor lymphocytes, preventing transfusion-associated GVHD in immunocompromised recipients. This modification is critical in early post-transplant care when immune recovery is incomplete. Other options address unrelated transfusion issues.
SubChapter: Hematologic and Transfusion Support

Q386. Answer: A

Explanation: Posaconazole provides broad antifungal coverage, including Aspergillus species, during prolonged neutropenia or GVHD. Acyclovir and ganciclovir target viruses, while ciprofloxacin covers bacteria. Extended prophylaxis reduces invasive fungal infection rates.
SubChapter: Infection Prevention and Management

Q387. Answer: A

Explanation: Cytokine release syndrome results from early, robust immune activation following mismatched or T-cell–replete grafts. It manifests as fever, hypotension, and hypoxia from IL-6 surge. Chronic GVHD and tumor lysis occur later in recovery.
SubChapter: Immune Reconstitution

Q388. Answer: D

Explanation: Acute GVHD typically manifests within 100 days after allogeneic transplant, presenting with jaundice (liver), diarrhea (gut), and rash (skin) due to donor T-cell attack on host tissues. Chronic GVHD occurs later, and CMV infection lacks this tri-organ involvement pattern.
SubChapter: Acute GVHD

Q389. Answer: A

Explanation: CMV reactivation risk is greatest in seropositive recipients receiving cells from seronegative donors because the virus persists latently and reactivates during immunosuppression. Autologous and cord blood transplants have significantly lower CMV risk due to reduced viral reservoir or delayed reactivation kinetics.
SubChapter: Infection Prevention and Management

Q390. Answer: A

Explanation: During neutrophil recovery, cytokine surges trigger sterile fevers, defining engraftment syndrome. It results from rapid immune reconstitution rather than infection. Transfusion and drug reactions are less frequent and present differently. Recognition prevents unnecessary antimicrobial escalation.
SubChapter: Immune Reconstitution

Q391. Answer: A

Explanation: Meticulous oral hygiene using gentle saline rinses prevents bacterial colonization and bloodstream invasion from mucosal breaks. This simple measure is highly effective in sepsis prevention. Restricting antibiotics or consuming raw foods increases infection risk during neutropenia.
SubChapter: Sepsis Management

Q392. Answer: D

Explanation: The liver is the primary target of veno-occlusive disease due to endothelial injury from conditioning regimens, leading to congestion, hepatomegaly, and hyperbilirubinemia. Other organs can be secondarily affected by hepatic dysfunction and fluid overload.
SubChapter: Acute System-Specific Complications

Q393. Answer: A

Explanation: A rising CMV viral load by polymerase chain reaction (PCR) identifies early reactivation before symptoms occur. This allows timely initiation of antiviral therapy, preventing pneumonitis or colitis. Other labs are nonspecific or unrelated to viral replication.
SubChapter: Infection Prevention and Management

Q394. Answer: A

Explanation: Neutropenic diets exclude raw or undercooked foods to prevent ingestion of pathogens while gut mucosa remains compromised. Emphasis is placed on safe food handling and fully cooked meals. Nutrient restriction is unnecessary unless indicated by other conditions.
SubChapter: Nutritional Support

Q395. Answer: A

Explanation: Engraftment syndrome arises during marrow recovery and features fever, erythematous rash, and noninfectious pulmonary infiltrates due to cytokine release. Absence of microbial growth distinguishes it from sepsis. Jaundice and diarrhea suggest GVHD or hepatic complications.
SubChapter: Immune Reconstitution

Q396. Answer: D

Explanation: Acyclovir effectively prevents herpes simplex and varicella-zoster reactivation during immunosuppression. It is administered orally or intravenously through immune recovery. Other listed agents target bacteria or fungi and are ineffective against HSV.
SubChapter: Infection Prevention and Management

Q397. Answer: A

Explanation: Both conditions may present with fever and hypotension, but sepsis is identified by positive cultures confirming microbial infection. Cytokine release syndrome produces sterile inflammatory findings, requiring IL-6 blockade rather than antibiotics.
SubChapter: Sepsis Management

Q398. Answer: A

Explanation: Tissue biopsy provides histologic confirmation of GVHD, revealing lymphocytic infiltration and epithelial apoptosis. Laboratory findings and cultures assist differential diagnosis but cannot confirm immune-mediated tissue injury. Biopsy guides targeted immunosuppressive therapy.
SubChapter: Acute GVHD

Q399. Answer: A

Explanation: HEPA-filtered environments minimize airborne fungal spores, particularly Aspergillus, during neutropenia. Environmental control is vital in transplant units. Probiotics and supplements do not prevent invasive fungal infections and may pose contamination risks.
SubChapter: Infection Prevention and Management

Q400. Answer: D

Explanation: Amphotericin B induces renal tubular wasting of potassium and magnesium, necessitating close electrolyte monitoring. Hypokalemia increases arrhythmia risk during therapy. Sodium and calcium levels typically remain stable. Supplementation and hydration mitigate toxicity.
SubChapter: Infection Prevention and Management

Questions (401-500)

Q401. Which early manifestation is characteristic of sepsis in immunocompromised patients?

A. Unexplained fever
B. Elevated white blood cell count
C. Productive cough
D. Skin rash

Q402. What is the preferred management of mild hepatic veno-occlusive disease?

A. Supportive care and ursodiol
B. High-dose corticosteroids
C. Antithymocyte globulin
D. Plasma exchange

Q403. Which blood product is safest for transfusion immediately after allogeneic transplant?

A. Irradiated and leukoreduced red blood cells
B. Fresh whole blood
C. Non-irradiated platelets
D. Cryoprecipitate without processing

Q404. What is the most common cause of early post-transplant mortality aside from infection?

A. Relapse of disease
B. Chronic GVHD
C. Secondary malignancy
D. Multi-organ failure from conditioning toxicity

Q405. What is the recommended first-line treatment for bacterial sepsis in neutropenic transplant patients?

A. Broad-spectrum intravenous antibiotics
B. Oral antibiotics
C. Corticosteroids
D. Observation until cultures return

Q406. Which measure best supports immune recovery following engraftment?

A. Adherence to antimicrobial prophylaxis and vaccination schedule
B. Discontinuation of immunosuppressants early
C. Daily exercise only
D. Avoidance of blood transfusion

Q407. Which post-transplant infection is primarily prevented through vaccination after immune recovery?

A. Streptococcus pneumoniae
B. Cytomegalovirus
C. Candida albicans
D. Aspergillus fumigatus

Q408. A transplant recipient develops fever and rash during neutrophil recovery. Cultures are negative, and symptoms improve with corticosteroids. What is the most likely diagnosis?

A. Drug hypersensitivity
B. Acute GVHD
C. CMV reactivation
D. Engraftment syndrome

Q409. Which laboratory test best detects early fungal infection in post-transplant patients?

A. Serum galactomannan assay
B. CMV PCR

C. Blood culture
D. Urinalysis

Q410. What is the primary action when tacrolimus trough level exceeds target range?
A. Hold the next dose and notify the provider
B. Administer extra hydration
C. Increase steroid therapy
D. Continue same dose until symptoms occur

Q411. Which condition presents with elevated bilirubin, right upper quadrant pain, and ascites after high-dose chemotherapy?
A. Veno-occlusive disease
B. Hepatic GVHD
C. Sepsis
D. Cytokine release syndrome

Q412. What symptom combination is most characteristic of acute GVHD?
A. Petechiae and pallor
B. Fever and neutropenia
C. Cough and dyspnea
D. Rash, diarrhea, and jaundice

Q413. Which supportive care strategy is most effective for patients with severe mucositis?
A. Parenteral nutrition
B. Mouth rinses with alcohol-based solutions
C. Discontinuation of fluids
D. Oral multivitamins only

Q414. Which type of infection is most likely during the first 30 days after allogeneic transplant?
A. Bacterial sepsis
B. CMV pneumonitis
C. Fungal sinusitis
D. Herpes zoster

Q415. A patient develops tremor and hypertension while on cyclosporine. What does this indicate?
A. Drug toxicity
B. Early sepsis
C. GVHD progression
D. Magnesium deficiency

Q416. Which antifungal is preferred for Aspergillus prophylaxis in high-risk GVHD patients?
A. Caspofungin
B. Fluconazole
C. Amphotericin B
D. Posaconazole

Q417. What finding best indicates immune reconstitution after allogeneic transplant?
A. Gradual rise in lymphocyte count
B. Return of appetite
C. Normal bilirubin
D. Stable platelet count

Q418. What intervention is critical for preventing infection-related mortality during neutropenia?
A. Immediate empiric antibiotic therapy with fever
B. Early taper of immunosuppression
C. Avoidance of all visitors
D. Routine viral testing

Q419. What complication is most closely linked to high-dose busulfan conditioning?
A. Hepatic veno-occlusive disease
B. Renal failure
C. Peripheral neuropathy
D. Cataract formation
Q420. Which action prevents bacterial infections originating from central lines post-transplant?
A. Covering dressing continuously without change
B. Routine heparin flush every hour
C. Immediate line removal at discharge
D. Strict aseptic line care and daily site assessment
Q421. A transplant patient's blood pressure rises while on tacrolimus. What mechanism explains this effect?
A. Renal vasoconstriction and sodium retention
B. Volume depletion
C. Adrenal suppression
D. Increased diuresis
Q422. What symptom requires urgent evaluation in a post-transplant patient?
A. Fever above 38°C
B. Mild fatigue
C. Loss of appetite
D. Hair thinning
Q423. What therapy is effective for steroid-refractory chronic GVHD but occasionally used for acute cases?
A. Extracorporeal photopheresis
B. Methotrexate
C. Levofloxacin
D. Amphotericin B
Q424. Which clinical sign suggests severe sepsis rather than localized infection?
A. Mild tachycardia
B. Single-site erythema
C. Oral ulcers
D. Hypotension unresponsive to fluids
Q425. What dietary recommendation supports hematologic recovery after transplant?
A. High-protein, calorie-dense foods
B. Low-sodium diet
C. Vegan-only meals
D. Restriction of fats
Q426. What is the purpose of leukoreduction in blood products for transplant recipients?
A. Reduce febrile reactions and CMV transmission
B. Prevent GVHD
C. Extend shelf life
D. Reduce hemolysis
Q427. What teaching should nurses emphasize before patient discharge after stem cell transplant?
A. Monitor temperature daily and report fever immediately
B. Resume all previous medications
C. Stop prophylactic antimicrobials when feeling well
D. Attend large gatherings to regain normalcy
Q428. Which laboratory trend confirms platelet engraftment?

A. Rising bilirubin levels
B. ANC >500 for one day
C. Platelet count >20,000/µL for three days without transfusion
D. Stable hemoglobin for a week

Q429. What infection risk is highest between day 30 and 100 post-transplant?
A. CMV reactivation
B. Bacterial sepsis
C. Fungal sinusitis
D. HSV reactivation

Q430. A patient develops painful oral ulcers after chemotherapy. What is the most appropriate nursing action?
A. Encourage saline and sodium bicarbonate rinses
B. Use hydrogen peroxide mouthwash
C. Allow dry mouth to form scabs
D. Provide acidic drinks to clean mucosa

Q431. What is the major side effect of high-dose corticosteroids for GVHD?
A. Hyperglycemia and muscle wasting
B. Nephrotoxicity
C. Hearing loss
D. Bradycardia

Q432. What complication results from donor immune cells attacking host tissues?
A. Tumor lysis
B. Graft rejection
C. Engraftment syndrome
D. GVHD

Q433. Which patient care measure prevents central-line infections in neutropenic patients?
A. Daily sterile dressing changes and site assessment
B. Using nonsterile gloves for quick checks
C. Avoiding flushing to reduce infection
D. Leaving dressings unchanged until discharge

Q434. A patient on cyclosporine has creatinine rising to 2.0 mg/dL. What should the nurse do first?
A. Hold the dose and notify the provider
B. Administer furosemide
C. Encourage oral fluids only
D. Continue and monitor tomorrow

Q435. Which action reduces the risk of veno-occlusive disease in transplant patients?
A. Administer ursodiol as prophylaxis
B. Restrict oral intake
C. Increase steroid dose
D. Delay conditioning therapy

Q436. What intervention helps prevent Pneumocystis jirovecii pneumonia after transplant?
A. Acyclovir prophylaxis
B. Fluconazole prophylaxis
C. Trimethoprim-sulfamethoxazole prophylaxis
D. Avoidance of live vaccines

Q437. What finding indicates possible sepsis in a post-transplant patient?
A. Fever and hypotension
B. Constipation

C. Weight gain
D. Hair loss

Q438. Which antifungal agent provides prophylaxis against both Candida and Aspergillus?
A. Posaconazole
B. Fluconazole
C. Amphotericin B
D. Terbinafine

Q439. A patient develops watery diarrhea on day +25 post-transplant. Which test confirms diagnosis of GI GVHD?
A. Colon biopsy
B. Stool culture
C. CT scan
D. CBC

Q440. What is the primary goal of infection prophylaxis during neutropenia?
A. Eliminate all pathogens
B. Maintain gut flora balance
C. Prevent microbial colonization and bloodstream invasion
D. Avoid broad-spectrum antibiotic resistance

Q441. What complication may develop if immunosuppressants are abruptly discontinued post-transplant?
A. Acute GVHD
B. Sepsis
C. Engraftment failure
D. Hypomagnesemia

Q442. Which laboratory change confirms immune reconstitution?
A. Gradual rise in lymphocyte subsets
B. Mild anemia improvement
C. Decline in bilirubin
D. Increase in creatinine

Q443. What is the most frequent cause of early post-transplant mortality?
A. Infection leading to sepsis
B. Chronic GVHD
C. Disease relapse
D. Graft rejection

Q444. Which nursing action prevents fungal infections in neutropenic patients?
A. Reduce antifungal prophylaxis
B. Limit showering to once weekly
C. Encourage raw fruit intake
D. Avoid potted plants and standing water in rooms

Q445. What symptom combination suggests hepatic GVHD?
A. Elevated bilirubin, alkaline phosphatase, and hepatomegaly
B. Fever and rash only
C. Hypotension and ascites
D. Weight loss and neutropenia

Q446. What patient education should be emphasized before discharge after transplant?
A. Avoid crowded areas and report fever immediately
B. Stop antivirals once appetite returns
C. Drink unboiled water for hydration

D. Visit family gatherings regularly

Q447. Which complication results from rapid cytokine release after donor lymphocyte infusion?

A. Cytokine release syndrome
B. Chronic GVHD
C. Engraftment failure
D. Tumor lysis syndrome

Q448. A patient 3 weeks post-transplant presents with watery diarrhea and skin rash. Which is the most likely diagnosis?

A. CMV colitis
B. Engraftment syndrome
C. Acute GVHD
D. Bacterial enteritis

Q449. Which preventive measure best reduces risk of bacterial infection during neutropenia?

A. Oral ciprofloxacin prophylaxis
B. Routine vitamin C supplementation
C. Limiting oral fluids
D. Topical antiseptics only

Q450. A patient on tacrolimus reports tremors and headache. Which lab finding would confirm drug toxicity?

A. Elevated tacrolimus trough level
B. Decreased magnesium
C. Low creatinine
D. Elevated bilirubin

Q451. Which of the following indicates successful neutrophil engraftment?

A. ANC >500 for three consecutive days
B. Platelet count >50,000/µL
C. Hemoglobin >12 g/dL
D. Normal bilirubin levels

Q452. Which organism most frequently causes bloodstream infections in neutropenic patients?

A. CMV
B. Aspergillus fumigatus
C. Candida albicans
D. Pseudomonas aeruginosa

Q453. Which intervention is essential for managing sepsis in transplant patients?

A. Immediate empiric IV antibiotics
B. Oral rehydration therapy
C. Observation for 24 hours
D. Delay antibiotics until culture results

Q454. What finding distinguishes hepatic GVHD from veno-occlusive disease?

A. Timing and enzyme pattern
B. Presence of ascites
C. Weight gain
D. Fever

Q455. Which action prevents Pneumocystis jirovecii pneumonia in immunocompromised patients?

A. Prophylaxis with trimethoprim-sulfamethoxazole
B. Prophylaxis with fluconazole
C. Early steroid taper
D. Vaccination with inactivated virus

Q456. Which complication should be suspected in a patient with fever, rash, and pulmonary infiltrates unresponsive to antibiotics?
A. CMV pneumonia
B. Bacterial sepsis
C. Chronic GVHD
D. Engraftment syndrome
Q457. Which symptom combination indicates early sepsis?
A. Fever, tachycardia, and hypotension
B. Weight gain and edema
C. Rash and itching
D. Nausea and vomiting
Q458. Which antifungal is preferred for prolonged prophylaxis in patients with chronic GVHD?
A. Posaconazole
B. Fluconazole
C. Amphotericin B
D. Terbinafine
Q459. Which electrolyte abnormalities are common in patients on calcineurin inhibitors?
A. Hyperkalemia and hypomagnesemia
B. Hypocalcemia
C. Hypernatremia
D. Hyponatremia
Q460. Which nursing intervention minimizes infection risk from mucositis?
A. Applying topical anesthetic only
B. Using hydrogen peroxide rinses
C. Avoiding oral care until mucosa heals
D. Frequent gentle mouth rinsing with saline
Q461. A patient develops hyperbilirubinemia and ascites 2 weeks post-conditioning. Which complication is suspected?
A. Veno-occlusive disease
B. Acute GVHD
C. Sepsis
D. Hepatic infection
Q462. Which laboratory parameter is monitored to evaluate CMV prophylaxis effectiveness?
A. CMV PCR viral load
B. White blood cell count
C. C-reactive protein
D. Total bilirubin
Q463. Which patient education is most important after hospital discharge?
A. Check temperature daily and report fever >38°C
B. Resume raw food diet
C. Limit oral hydration
D. Discontinue antivirals when appetite improves
Q464. What clinical feature differentiates acute GVHD from engraftment syndrome?
A. Fever
B. Presence of rash
C. Timing after transplant
D. Pulmonary infiltrates
Q465. Which intervention prevents transfusion-associated GVHD?

A. Irradiation of blood products
B. Leukoreduction alone
C. Washing red blood cells
D. Cryopreservation of plasma

Q466. Which infection typically develops during late post-transplant recovery (>100 days)?
A. Community-acquired respiratory infections
B. Bacterial sepsis
C. CMV reactivation
D. Early fungal pneumonia

Q467. What patient education should be reinforced regarding immunosuppressant adherence?
A. Never skip doses or adjust medication without provider approval
B. Stop therapy when symptoms improve
C. Double doses if one is missed
D. Take with grapefruit juice for absorption

Q468. Which symptom combination suggests early acute GVHD?
A. Dry mouth and joint pain
B. Hypotension, fever, and confusion
C. Maculopapular rash, diarrhea, and elevated bilirubin
D. Cough and nasal congestion

Q469. What is the most effective infection control measure for immunocompromised inpatients?
A. Strict hand hygiene
B. Routine mask use by staff only
C. Private room with closed door
D. Limited bathing frequency

Q470. A patient receiving total parenteral nutrition develops fever and positive blood cultures for Staphylococcus epidermidis. What is the likely source?
A. Central venous catheter
B. Contaminated parenteral solution
C. Oral mucositis
D. Urinary tract infection

Q471. Which patient is most at risk for fungal pneumonia post-transplant?
A. Allogeneic recipient with prolonged neutropenia
B. Autologous recipient on day +7
C. Patient post-engraftment with stable counts
D. Donor prior to stem cell harvest

Q472. What early complication results from cytokine-mediated capillary leak during engraftment?
A. Acute GVHD
B. Veno-occlusive disease
C. Engraftment syndrome
D. Cardiac tamponade

Q473. Which immunosuppressant requires level monitoring to prevent nephrotoxicity?
A. Tacrolimus
B. Methotrexate
C. Cyclophosphamide
D. Azathioprine

Q474. A transplant patient presents with jaundice, right upper quadrant pain, and weight gain. Which condition should be suspected?
A. Veno-occlusive disease

B. Hepatic GVHD
C. CMV hepatitis
D. Bacterial cholangitis

Q475. Which prophylactic agent prevents herpes simplex virus reactivation?
A. Acyclovir
B. Fluconazole
C. Levofloxacin
D. Amphotericin B

Q476. What is the best indicator of hematologic recovery after stem cell transplant?
A. Stable neutrophil and platelet counts
B. Normal bilirubin
C. Improved appetite
D. Decreased creatinine

Q477. What electrolyte imbalance is common with amphotericin B therapy?
A. Hyponatremia
B. Hypercalcemia
C. Hypokalemia and hypomagnesemia
D. Hyperkalemia

Q478. What immediate nursing action is indicated for a febrile neutropenic patient?
A. Obtain cultures and start empiric antibiotics
B. Observe temperature trend for one hour
C. Begin corticosteroid therapy
D. Administer antifungal prophylaxis only

Q479. Which late infection is prevented through vaccination post-transplant?
A. Streptococcus pneumoniae
B. CMV
C. Candida albicans
D. Aspergillus fumigatus

Q480. A patient develops hypertension and elevated creatinine on cyclosporine. What should the nurse suspect?
A. Drug toxicity
B. Acute GVHD
C. Sepsis
D. Hypovolemia

Q481. What condition causes noninfectious fever and pulmonary infiltrates during engraftment?
A. Bacterial sepsis
B. CMV pneumonia
C. Engraftment syndrome
D. Chronic GVHD

Q482. What nursing action supports prevention of fungal infections?
A. Maintain HEPA filtration in patient rooms
B. Use humidifiers daily
C. Encourage visitors with masks
D. Avoid cleaning air vents

Q483. What is the leading cause of death during the first month after transplant?
A. Infection-related sepsis
B. Chronic GVHD
C. Disease relapse

D. Secondary malignancy

Q484. Which nursing instruction is vital for a patient starting immunosuppressants?

A. Report fever, rash, or tremors immediately
B. Stop medication during mild nausea
C. Avoid all vaccinations
D. Take doses only on alternate days

Q485. What dietary advice supports recovery post-transplant?

A. Follow a raw vegetable diet
B. Include unpasteurized dairy
C. Consume high-protein, cooked foods only
D. Avoid all carbohydrates

Q486. Which blood product modification prevents CMV transmission?

A. Leukoreduction
B. Irradiation
C. Cryopreservation
D. Washing

Q487. A 48-year-old allogeneic HSCT survivor reports persistent dry eyes and oral ulcers six months post-transplant. Which complication should the nurse suspect?

A. Cytomegalovirus reactivation
B. Chronic graft-versus-host disease
C. Iron overload
D. Secondary malignancy

Q488. A patient presents with exertional dyspnea and a nonproductive cough 18 months post-transplant. High-resolution CT reveals bronchiolitis obliterans. What is the initial management approach?

A. Broad-spectrum antibiotics
B. Corticosteroids and immunosuppression adjustment
C. Bronchodilators only
D. Observation

Q489. Which late endocrine effect is most commonly observed in adult HSCT survivors?

A. Hypothyroidism
B. Addison's disease
C. Hyperparathyroidism
D. Pheochromocytoma

Q490. A 35-year-old female survivor asks when she should resume vaccinations after allogeneic HSCT. What is the nurse's best response?

A. "Restart vaccines six months after transplant."
B. "Begin routine vaccines at 12 months post-transplant."
C. "Vaccines are unnecessary after engraftment."
D. "Resume childhood series at 24 months post-transplant."

Q491. What is the most effective strategy for preventing late cardiovascular complications in HSCT survivors?

A. Lifelong anticoagulation
B. Routine echocardiography every six months
C. Managing modifiable risk factors such as hypertension and dyslipidemia
D. Daily corticosteroid prophylaxis

Q492. A post-transplant patient presents with chronic skin sclerosis and joint stiffness. What long-term complication is indicated?

A. Sclerodermatous chronic GVHD
B. Autoimmune thyroiditis
C. Iron overload arthropathy
D. Gout

Q493. Which long-term renal complication can result from calcineurin inhibitor therapy post-HSCT?

A. Nephrotic syndrome
B. Chronic nephrotoxicity leading to hypertension
C. Hypokalemia
D. Nephrolithiasis

Q494. Which symptom requires urgent evaluation for possible secondary malignancy in a long-term HSCT survivor?

A. Fatigue
B. Unexplained lymphadenopathy
C. Joint pain
D. Oral dryness

Q495. Which teaching point best supports late infection prevention in chronic GVHD patients?

A. Avoid outdoor activity
B. Discontinue antimicrobial prophylaxis early
C. Maintain up-to-date vaccinations and prompt infection reporting
D. Rely on herbal supplements

Q496. A 50-year-old autologous transplant survivor develops bone pain and osteopenia five years post-treatment. What is the most likely cause?

A. Vitamin D deficiency
B. Steroid-induced osteoporosis
C. Paraneoplastic syndrome
D. Iron overload

Q497. What is the recommended screening for secondary skin cancers after HSCT?

A. Annual full-body skin exam
B. Monthly self-exam only
C. Screening only if lesions appear
D. No routine screening

Q498. A patient on long-term corticosteroids post-HSCT experiences mood swings and insomnia. What nursing intervention is appropriate?

A. Taper steroid dose independently
B. Encourage sleep hygiene and coordinate psychiatric evaluation
C. Double steroid dose temporarily
D. Discontinue immunosuppressants immediately

Q499. Which of the following nutritional strategies is most appropriate for long-term HSCT survivors?

A. High-iron diet
B. Balanced diet emphasizing protein and calcium
C. Low-protein diet
D. Strict carbohydrate restriction

Q500. A patient asks about fertility recovery two years post-transplant. The nurse explains that:

A. Most regain fertility within six months.
B. Fertility recovery depends on conditioning regimen intensity and sex.
C. Transplant guarantees permanent infertility.
D. Recovery occurs only after ten years.

Answer key and Explanation (401-500)

Q401. Answer: A

Explanation: Fever may be the only early indicator of sepsis in immunocompromised patients due to blunted inflammatory responses. Prompt recognition and empiric antibiotic initiation prevent rapid progression to septic shock.

SubChapter: Sepsis Management

Q402. Answer: A

Explanation: Supportive measures including fluid restriction, diuretics, and ursodiol help reduce hepatic congestion in mild VOD. Severe cases may require defibrotide. Corticosteroids and plasma exchange are ineffective and potentially harmful.

SubChapter: Acute System-Specific Complications

Q403. Answer: A

Explanation: Irradiated and leukoreduced red cells prevent transfusion-associated GVHD and febrile reactions in immunocompromised recipients. Whole blood and non-processed components carry high immune risk. This modification is standard during early recovery.

SubChapter: Hematologic and Transfusion Support

Q404. Answer: D

Explanation: Intensive conditioning regimens can cause early organ toxicity leading to multi-organ failure, second only to infection as a cause of early mortality. Chronic GVHD and relapse typically occur months later during immune recovery.

SubChapter: Acute System-Specific Complications

Q405. Answer: A

Explanation: Immediate empiric broad-spectrum IV antibiotics are critical in neutropenic sepsis to cover gram-negative and gram-positive bacteria. Delayed or oral therapy risks rapid clinical deterioration. Culture results refine subsequent therapy.

SubChapter: Sepsis Management

Q406. Answer: A

Explanation: Consistent adherence to antimicrobial prophylaxis and scheduled vaccinations ensures safe immune reconstitution while minimizing infection risk. Early cessation of immunosuppression can trigger GVHD, and lifestyle measures alone cannot replace medical protection.

SubChapter: Immune Reconstitution

Q407. Answer: A

Explanation: Vaccination against Streptococcus pneumoniae and other encapsulated bacteria is vital once immune recovery allows, preventing late bacterial infections. CMV and fungal pathogens require antiviral and antifungal prophylaxis, not vaccination.

SubChapter: Infection Prevention and Management

Q408. Answer: D

Explanation: Engraftment syndrome occurs during neutrophil recovery due to cytokine release, presenting as fever, rash, and pulmonary symptoms without infection. It responds rapidly to corticosteroids, unlike GVHD, which involves tissue-specific immune injury and slower improvement.

SubChapter: Immune Reconstitution

Q409. Answer: A

Explanation: The serum galactomannan assay identifies Aspergillus antigen before radiologic changes, allowing earlier antifungal therapy. Blood cultures rarely detect fungi in neutropenic patients. CMV PCR and urinalysis screen for unrelated infections.

SubChapter: Infection Prevention and Management

Q410. Answer: A

Explanation: Elevated tacrolimus levels can cause nephrotoxicity and neurotoxicity. Holding the medication and notifying the provider allows for dose adjustment. Hydration may support renal function but does not replace clinical intervention.
SubChapter: Immunosuppressive Therapy

Q411. Answer: A

Explanation: Veno-occlusive disease results from hepatic sinusoidal obstruction following conditioning therapy, producing jaundice, pain, and fluid retention. Hepatic GVHD appears later and presents differently. Early management with defibrotide improves survival outcomes.
SubChapter: Acute System-Specific Complications

Q412. Answer: D

Explanation: Acute GVHD typically affects skin, GI tract, and liver, producing rash, diarrhea, and hyperbilirubinemia. These signs represent systemic donor T-cell activity. Other symptoms indicate infection or hematologic issues, not GVHD.
SubChapter: Acute GVHD

Q413. Answer: A

Explanation: Parenteral nutrition provides adequate caloric and protein support when oral intake is impaired by mucositis. Alcohol-based rinses worsen pain, and fluid restriction exacerbates dehydration. Early nutrition support promotes mucosal healing.
SubChapter: Nutritional Support

Q414. Answer: A

Explanation: Early post-transplant infections are predominantly bacterial due to mucosal barrier disruption and neutropenia. Viral and fungal infections appear later as immunosuppression persists. Early empiric antibiotic therapy is essential to prevent mortality.
SubChapter: Infection Prevention and Management

Q415. Answer: A

Explanation: Cyclosporine toxicity manifests as tremor, hypertension, and nephrotoxicity. Monitoring drug levels and renal function prevents irreversible injury. Sepsis and GVHD have distinct systemic signs, and magnesium deficiency alone does not cause hypertension.
SubChapter: Immunosuppressive Therapy

Q416. Answer: D

Explanation: Posaconazole provides extended mold coverage including Aspergillus, making it superior for GVHD patients receiving prolonged immunosuppression. Fluconazole lacks mold activity, and amphotericin B has higher toxicity. Caspofungin is reserved for treatment, not prophylaxis.
SubChapter: Infection Prevention and Management

Q417. Answer: A

Explanation: Lymphocyte recovery signifies adaptive immune reconstitution, marking restoration of donor-derived immunity. While other parameters reflect clinical stability, lymphocyte increase directly correlates with immune competence and reduced infection risk.
SubChapter: Immune Reconstitution

Q418. Answer: A

Explanation: Empiric antibiotic initiation at the first fever sign significantly reduces mortality in neutropenic patients. Visitor restrictions and viral screening help but cannot replace rapid antimicrobial coverage for potential bacterial sepsis.
SubChapter: Sepsis Management

Q419. Answer: A

Explanation: Busulfan damages hepatic endothelium, predisposing to veno-occlusive disease with jaundice and fluid retention. Renal and neurologic effects are less common. Dose monitoring and ursodiol prophylaxis reduce hepatic complications.

SubChapter: Acute System-Specific Complications

Q420. Answer: D

Explanation: Aseptic central line maintenance and regular inspection prevent catheter-related bloodstream infections. Frequent heparin use or static dressings increase risk. Proper dressing changes and sterile technique are vital during neutropenia.

SubChapter: Infection Prevention and Management

Q421. Answer: A

Explanation: Tacrolimus causes renal vasoconstriction and sodium retention, elevating blood pressure. This effect mirrors cyclosporine toxicity and warrants dose review. Adrenal suppression or dehydration are unrelated to this mechanism.

SubChapter: Immunosuppressive Therapy

Q422. Answer: A

Explanation: Fever in an immunocompromised transplant recipient is a medical emergency suggesting potential sepsis. Prompt cultures and empiric antibiotics prevent rapid deterioration. Other symptoms may reflect recovery or medication side effects but are not emergent.

SubChapter: Sepsis Management

Q423. Answer: A

Explanation: Extracorporeal photopheresis modulates T-cell activity, improving steroid-refractory chronic GVHD and selected acute GVHD cases. It offers immunomodulatory benefits without severe systemic toxicity. The other agents serve unrelated prophylactic or antimicrobial roles.

SubChapter: Acute GVHD

Q424. Answer: D

Explanation: Refractory hypotension indicates septic shock from systemic inflammatory response and circulatory failure. It distinguishes severe sepsis from localized infections. Immediate hemodynamic support and broad antibiotics are required to prevent organ failure.

SubChapter: Sepsis Management

Q425. Answer: A

Explanation: Protein and calorie-rich nutrition promotes hematopoietic regeneration, immune reconstitution, and wound healing post-transplant. Restrictive or unbalanced diets limit marrow recovery and delay engraftment. Early nutritional optimization supports recovery.

SubChapter: Nutritional Support

Q426. Answer: A

Explanation: Leukoreduction filters donor leukocytes, reducing febrile nonhemolytic transfusion reactions and CMV transmission. Irradiation, not leukoreduction, prevents GVHD. These modifications enhance transfusion safety for immunocompromised patients.

SubChapter: Hematologic and Transfusion Support

Q427. Answer: A

Explanation: Daily temperature monitoring allows early infection detection, enabling prompt treatment and preventing sepsis. Stopping prophylaxis or exposure to crowds increases infection risk. Reinforcing vigilance ensures post-discharge safety and graft success.

SubChapter: Patient and Caregiver Education

Q428. Answer: C

Explanation: Platelet engraftment is defined as a sustained platelet count above 20,000/μL for three consecutive days without transfusion support. This indicates successful megakaryocytic recovery and donor marrow function. Hemoglobin and ANC values assess other hematopoietic lines.

SubChapter: Hematologic and Immune Reconstitution

Q429. Answer: A

Explanation: CMV reactivation typically occurs during the intermediate phase (day 30–100) when cellular immunity is recovering but incomplete. Early bacterial sepsis predominates before engraftment, and HSV reactivation is usually prevented by antiviral prophylaxis.
SubChapter: Infection Prevention and Management

Q430. Answer: A

Explanation: Saline or sodium bicarbonate rinses soothe mucosal irritation, prevent infection, and promote healing in chemotherapy-induced ulcers. Hydrogen peroxide and acidic fluids worsen mucosal breakdown and pain. Hydration and oral care are critical in neutropenia management.
SubChapter: Nutritional Support

Q431. Answer: A

Explanation: Corticosteroids commonly cause hyperglycemia, muscle wasting, mood changes, and immunosuppression. These effects require glucose monitoring and infection vigilance. Nephrotoxicity and bradycardia are unrelated to steroid mechanisms.
SubChapter: Acute GVHD

Q432. Answer: D

Explanation: GVHD occurs when donor T-cells recognize host tissues as foreign, leading to multisystem inflammation, particularly in the skin, liver, and GI tract. Graft rejection involves host immunity, while engraftment syndrome stems from cytokine activation.
SubChapter: Acute GVHD

Q433. Answer: A

Explanation: Strict aseptic technique and daily assessment reduce bloodstream infection risk from central venous lines. Regular dressing changes prevent bacterial colonization. Neglect or poor technique greatly increases mortality during neutropenia.
SubChapter: Infection Prevention and Management

Q434. Answer: A

Explanation: Rising creatinine under cyclosporine suggests nephrotoxicity. Holding the dose and notifying the provider prevents permanent renal damage. Adjustments or substitution may be required. Supportive measures alone are insufficient without intervention.
SubChapter: Immunosuppressive Therapy

Q435. Answer: A

Explanation: Ursodiol stabilizes bile flow and protects hepatic endothelial cells, reducing veno-occlusive disease risk. Nutritional restriction and steroid escalation offer no preventive benefit. Early prophylaxis is standard for high-risk regimens.
SubChapter: Acute System-Specific Complications

Q436. Answer: C

Explanation: TMP-SMX is the first-line prophylactic for Pneumocystis jirovecii infection. It effectively prevents opportunistic pneumonia in immunocompromised patients. Fluconazole and acyclovir target fungi and viruses, respectively, and do not cover this organism.
SubChapter: Infection Prevention and Management

Q437. Answer: A

Explanation: Fever and hypotension in an immunocompromised patient signal sepsis until proven otherwise. Immediate evaluation and empiric antibiotic initiation are required to prevent organ failure. Other symptoms are noninfectious and not emergent.
SubChapter: Sepsis Management

Q438. Answer: A

Explanation: Posaconazole has broad antifungal coverage, including molds like Aspergillus and yeasts such as Candida, making it ideal for high-risk transplant patients. Fluconazole lacks mold activity, and amphotericin B is more toxic for routine prophylaxis.

SubChapter: Infection Prevention and Management

Q439. Answer: A

Explanation: Colon biopsy provides histologic confirmation of GI GVHD, revealing apoptotic crypt cells and lymphocytic infiltration. Stool cultures rule out infection but cannot confirm immune-mediated injury. Imaging and CBC are nonspecific.

SubChapter: Acute GVHD

Q440. Answer: C

Explanation: Prophylactic antimicrobials and sterile practices aim to prevent microbial translocation and bloodstream infections during immune suppression. Complete pathogen elimination is unrealistic, but controlling exposure and colonization prevents sepsis.

SubChapter: Infection Prevention and Management

Q441. Answer: A

Explanation: Sudden withdrawal of immunosuppressive therapy can trigger acute GVHD due to unchecked donor T-cell activation. Gradual tapering under physician guidance is essential to maintain immune balance. Sepsis risk increases only indirectly from inflammation.

SubChapter: Immunosuppressive Therapy

Q442. Answer: A

Explanation: Immune reconstitution is confirmed by rising lymphocyte counts, particularly CD4 and CD8 cells, reflecting restored adaptive immunity. Other lab trends may reflect organ or hematologic recovery but not immune competence.

SubChapter: Immune Reconstitution

Q443. Answer: A

Explanation: Infections progressing to sepsis account for the majority of early transplant deaths due to severe neutropenia and mucosal barrier disruption. Chronic GVHD and relapse occur later, while graft rejection is less common in matched transplants.

SubChapter: Sepsis Management

Q444. Answer: D

Explanation: Environmental fungal control through avoidance of plants, soil, and stagnant water minimizes spore exposure, especially Aspergillus. Strict hygiene and consistent antifungal use further protect immunocompromised patients during neutropenia.

SubChapter: Infection Prevention and Management

Q445. Answer: A

Explanation: Hepatic GVHD manifests with cholestatic enzyme elevation and jaundice from bile duct inflammation by donor T-cells. Fever and rash indicate systemic involvement, but laboratory patterns confirm liver injury.

SubChapter: Acute GVHD

Q446. Answer: A

Explanation: Avoiding crowds and promptly reporting fever are vital infection-prevention strategies for recovering transplant patients. Prophylactic medications must continue as prescribed until immune recovery. Public exposure significantly raises infection risk.

SubChapter: Patient and Caregiver Education

Q447. Answer: A

Explanation: Cytokine release syndrome occurs when donor lymphocytes trigger massive cytokine production, leading to fever, hypotension, and hypoxia. It requires prompt recognition and IL-6 blockade. Chronic GVHD and engraftment failure arise later from different mechanisms.

SubChapter: Immune Reconstitution

Q448. Answer: C

Explanation: Acute GVHD occurs within 100 days post-transplant and typically presents with diarrhea, rash, and elevated bilirubin from immune-mediated tissue injury. Engraftment syndrome happens earlier and resolves quickly, while infectious causes usually have positive cultures or viral PCR results.
SubChapter: Acute GVHD

Q449. Answer: A

Explanation: Fluoroquinolone prophylaxis, such as ciprofloxacin, effectively reduces gram-negative bacterial infections in neutropenic patients. Vitamin supplements and topical antiseptics offer minimal systemic protection. Adequate hydration remains necessary to support renal function during antibiotic therapy.
SubChapter: Infection Prevention and Management

Q450. Answer: A

Explanation: Elevated tacrolimus trough levels confirm drug accumulation, explaining neurologic symptoms like tremors and headache. Monitoring blood levels prevents neuro- and nephrotoxicity. Magnesium loss may occur but is secondary to drug-induced renal changes.
SubChapter: Immunosuppressive Therapy

Q451. Answer: A

Explanation: Neutrophil engraftment, defined as ANC >500/mm^3 for three consecutive days, confirms functional bone marrow recovery. Platelet and hemoglobin normalization occur later. Liver function markers reflect unrelated organ health, not marrow reconstitution.
SubChapter: Hematologic and Immune Reconstitution

Q452. Answer: D

Explanation: Pseudomonas aeruginosa is a leading cause of bloodstream infections during neutropenia due to mucosal injury and central lines. Rapid empiric antipseudomonal coverage is crucial. Aspergillus and Candida are more common later or in persistent neutropenia.
SubChapter: Infection Prevention and Management

Q453. Answer: A

Explanation: Sepsis in immunocompromised patients requires prompt empiric IV antibiotics to prevent rapid progression to shock. Observation or delay significantly increases mortality. Broad-spectrum coverage is standard until cultures guide therapy adjustments.
SubChapter: Sepsis Management

Q454. Answer: A

Explanation: Hepatic GVHD typically appears later with cholestatic enzyme elevations, while VOD occurs early with hepatomegaly and weight gain. Timing and specific enzyme patterns help differentiate the two for targeted management.
SubChapter: Acute System-Specific Complications

Q455. Answer: A

Explanation: TMP-SMX effectively prevents Pneumocystis jirovecii infection, a life-threatening pneumonia in transplant patients. Antifungals and vaccines are ineffective for this organism, and early steroid tapering can increase GVHD risk.
SubChapter: Infection Prevention and Management

Q456. Answer: D

Explanation: Engraftment syndrome presents with fever, rash, and noninfectious pulmonary infiltrates during marrow recovery. Its sterile nature explains poor antibiotic response. Corticosteroids resolve symptoms quickly once infection is excluded.
SubChapter: Immune Reconstitution

Q457. Answer: A

Explanation: Early sepsis manifests as fever, tachycardia, and hypotension, reflecting systemic inflammatory response and poor perfusion. Immediate fluid resuscitation and broad-spectrum antibiotics are lifesaving. Other combinations indicate noninfectious conditions.
SubChapter: Sepsis Management

Q458. Answer: A

Explanation: Posaconazole offers broad coverage against yeasts and molds, making it ideal for patients with chronic GVHD who remain immunosuppressed. Fluconazole lacks mold activity, and amphotericin's toxicity limits long-term use.
SubChapter: Infection Prevention and Management

Q459. Answer: A

Explanation: Calcineurin inhibitors cause renal tubular dysfunction leading to potassium retention and magnesium wasting. Regular monitoring prevents arrhythmias and muscle weakness. Sodium and calcium changes are not typical with these drugs.
SubChapter: Immunosuppressive Therapy

Q460. Answer: D

Explanation: Regular saline rinsing reduces bacterial load and prevents sepsis from mucosal breaks. Hydrogen peroxide irritates tissue, and withholding oral care worsens infection risk. Topical anesthetics provide comfort but no antimicrobial effect.
SubChapter: Nutritional Support

Q461. Answer: A

Explanation: Veno-occlusive disease occurs within 21 days after conditioning, presenting with jaundice, hepatomegaly, and ascites from hepatic venous obstruction. Early detection allows intervention with defibrotide and supportive care.
SubChapter: Acute System-Specific Complications

Q462. Answer: A

Explanation: CMV PCR quantifies viral DNA, enabling early detection of reactivation and monitoring response to antiviral therapy. Other labs provide nonspecific inflammation or organ data but cannot track viral replication.
SubChapter: Infection Prevention and Management

Q463. Answer: A

Explanation: Daily temperature checks allow early detection of infection during ongoing immunosuppression. Immediate reporting of fever ensures timely management. Stopping prophylaxis or dietary neglect increases infection and dehydration risks.
SubChapter: Patient and Caregiver Education

Q464. Answer: C

Explanation: Timing distinguishes the two conditions: engraftment syndrome occurs during marrow recovery, while acute GVHD develops later after donor T-cell activation. Both can cause rash and fever, requiring histologic confirmation for GVHD.
SubChapter: Acute GVHD

Q465. Answer: A

Explanation: Irradiating blood products inactivates donor lymphocytes, preventing transfusion-associated GVHD in immunocompromised patients. Leukoreduction reduces reactions but not GVHD. Washing and cryopreservation serve different transfusion safety roles.
SubChapter: Hematologic and Transfusion Support

Q466. Answer: A

Explanation: As immune recovery progresses, patients become susceptible to community respiratory pathogens like influenza or RSV. Bacterial and fungal infections are more common earlier, and CMV reactivation usually occurs before full recovery.

SubChapter: Infection Prevention and Management

Q467. Answer: A

Explanation: Strict adherence to immunosuppressants prevents GVHD and graft failure. Patients must avoid self-adjustment or skipping doses. Grapefruit juice raises drug levels and toxicity risk. Clear education ensures stable immune control.

SubChapter: Immunosuppressive Therapy

Q468. Answer: C

Explanation: Acute GVHD commonly presents within 100 days post-transplant with skin rash, gastrointestinal symptoms, and hepatic dysfunction. These manifestations reflect immune-mediated tissue injury by donor lymphocytes. Chronic GVHD and infections occur later with distinct patterns.

SubChapter: Acute GVHD

Q469. Answer: A

Explanation: Rigorous hand hygiene is the most critical infection prevention practice, significantly reducing microbial transmission in immunocompromised patients. While isolation rooms and masks help, hand contact remains the predominant infection route in healthcare environments.

SubChapter: Infection Prevention and Management

Q470. Answer: A

Explanation: Central venous catheters are the most common source of Staphylococcus epidermidis bacteremia due to biofilm formation. Regular aseptic maintenance and prompt culture evaluation are essential. Contaminated TPN or mucositis rarely cause coagulase-negative staphylococcal infection.

SubChapter: Sepsis Management

Q471. Answer: A

Explanation: Prolonged neutropenia and allogeneic transplantation increase fungal pneumonia risk, especially from Aspergillus. Preventive measures include HEPA filtration and mold-active antifungal prophylaxis. Autologous transplants have lower infection risk due to shorter immunosuppression periods.

SubChapter: Infection Prevention and Management

Q472. Answer: C

Explanation: Engraftment syndrome causes fever, rash, and fluid retention from cytokine-induced endothelial injury during marrow recovery. It typically responds to corticosteroids and supportive care, distinguishing it from GVHD, which has histologic immune damage.

SubChapter: Immune Reconstitution

Q473. Answer: A

Explanation: Tacrolimus has a narrow therapeutic range, and elevated trough levels cause nephrotoxicity and neurotoxicity. Regular monitoring ensures efficacy without toxicity. Other agents have different toxicity profiles not routinely tracked by serum level testing.

SubChapter: Immunosuppressive Therapy

Q474. Answer: A

Explanation: Veno-occlusive disease occurs early post-transplant due to hepatic endothelial injury, leading to jaundice, hepatomegaly, and weight gain from fluid retention. GVHD presents later with cholestasis but lacks painful congestion.

SubChapter: Acute System-Specific Complications

Q475. Answer: A

Explanation: Acyclovir effectively prevents HSV reactivation during immunosuppression by inhibiting viral DNA synthesis. Antibacterial or antifungal drugs do not provide antiviral protection, highlighting the importance of tailored prophylaxis in transplant patients.

SubChapter: Infection Prevention and Management

Q476. Answer: A

Explanation: Rising neutrophil and platelet counts confirm marrow engraftment and hematologic recovery, signifying donor graft function. Other laboratory improvements indicate systemic stability but not direct marrow restoration.
SubChapter: Hematologic and Immune Reconstitution
Q477. Answer: C
Explanation: Amphotericin B causes renal tubular injury leading to potassium and magnesium loss. Monitoring and replacement are necessary during therapy to prevent cardiac and neuromuscular complications. Electrolyte surveillance ensures safe antifungal use.
SubChapter: Infection Prevention and Management
Q478. Answer: A
Explanation: In febrile neutropenia, early cultures and empiric broad-spectrum IV antibiotics are critical to prevent septic shock. Delay in therapy significantly increases mortality. Steroids and antifungals are adjuncts, not first-line measures.
SubChapter: Sepsis Management
Q479. Answer: A
Explanation: Vaccination against Streptococcus pneumoniae prevents life-threatening bacterial infections once immune recovery allows. Antiviral or antifungal prophylaxis addresses the others, as vaccines are not available or ineffective for those pathogens.
SubChapter: Infection Prevention and Management
Q480. Answer: A
Explanation: Cyclosporine-induced nephrotoxicity causes renal vasoconstriction, leading to elevated creatinine and hypertension. Early recognition prevents irreversible kidney injury through dose adjustment or substitution. Other causes show differing clinical contexts.
SubChapter: Immunosuppressive Therapy
Q481. Answer: C
Explanation: Engraftment syndrome results from immune reconstitution, causing fever, rash, and pulmonary infiltrates without infection. It responds to corticosteroids and supportive care. Infectious causes must be excluded before diagnosis.
SubChapter: Immune Reconstitution
Q482. Answer: A
Explanation: HEPA filtration removes airborne fungal spores such as Aspergillus, significantly lowering infection risk. Humidifiers and poor ventilation increase spore proliferation, and visitor traffic should be restricted during neutropenia.
SubChapter: Infection Prevention and Management
Q483. Answer: A
Explanation: Infection progressing to sepsis remains the primary cause of early mortality due to profound neutropenia and mucosal damage. Rapid diagnosis and empiric antibiotics are essential to improve survival during this high-risk period.
SubChapter: Sepsis Management
Q484. Answer: A
Explanation: Early reporting of fever, rash, or tremors helps detect infection or toxicity from immunosuppressants like tacrolimus or cyclosporine. Adherence and prompt communication prevent complications and maintain therapeutic balance.
SubChapter: Immunosuppressive Therapy
Q485. Answer: C
Explanation: High-protein, thoroughly cooked foods support immune recovery, tissue repair, and infection prevention. Raw or unpasteurized foods risk bacterial contamination during neutropenia. Balanced nutrition accelerates engraftment and healing.

SubChapter: Nutritional Support

Q486. Answer: A

Explanation: Leukoreduction removes donor leukocytes, reducing febrile reactions and CMV transmission risk. Irradiation prevents GVHD, while washing and cryopreservation serve other transfusion safety purposes. Leukoreduction is standard for immunocompromised patients.

SubChapter: Hematologic and Transfusion Support

Q487. Answer: B

Explanation: Chronic graft-versus-host disease often manifests with sicca symptoms like dry eyes and mouth due to immune-mediated mucosal inflammation. Option A is incorrect since CMV reactivation primarily causes systemic or pulmonary symptoms. Option C involves ferritin elevation and liver toxicity, not mucosal dryness. Option D develops years later, not within six months.

SubChapter: Late Post-Transplant Complications – Chronic GVHD

Q488. Answer: B

Explanation: Bronchiolitis obliterans is a late noninfectious pulmonary manifestation of chronic GVHD requiring corticosteroids and intensified immunosuppression. Option A is inappropriate unless infection is suspected. Option C may relieve symptoms but not control immune injury. Option D risks irreversible airway fibrosis without early intervention.

SubChapter: Pulmonary Late Effects – GVHD-related

Q489. Answer: A

Explanation: Hypothyroidism is the most frequent endocrine late effect, especially after total body irradiation or high-dose chemotherapy. Option B rarely follows HSCT. Option C is not typically related to transplant therapy. Option D occurs independently of transplant exposure.

SubChapter: Endocrine Late Effects

Q490. Answer: B

Explanation: Routine immunizations are reinitiated about 12 months post-transplant when immune reconstitution allows effective response. Option A is premature; immune function remains immature. Option C is unsafe due to susceptibility. Option D delays protection unnecessarily.

SubChapter: Long-Term Immune Reconstitution & Vaccination

Q491. Answer: C

Explanation: Controlling hypertension, dyslipidemia, and diabetes minimizes cardiotoxicity and metabolic syndrome linked to transplant therapy. Option A is not indicated universally. Option B is performed only when symptoms develop. Option D worsens risk by inducing metabolic derangements.

SubChapter: Late Cardiac Effects – Health Promotion

Q492. Answer: A

Explanation: Sclerodermatous chronic GVHD produces fibrotic skin tightening and contractures due to collagen deposition from immune activation. Option B affects the thyroid, not skin. Option C manifests with liver and joint iron accumulation but lacks skin sclerosis. Option D causes acute gouty inflammation, not chronic thickening.

SubChapter: Musculoskeletal & Dermatologic Late GVHD

Q493. Answer: B

Explanation: Calcineurin inhibitors such as cyclosporine or tacrolimus can cause chronic nephrotoxicity and hypertension due to renal vasoconstriction. Option A is rare. Option C results from diuretics, not immunosuppressants. Option D is unrelated to HSCT medication profiles.

SubChapter: Renal Late Effects

Q494. Answer: B

Explanation: New, persistent lymphadenopathy may indicate post-transplant lymphoproliferative disorder or secondary malignancy and warrants immediate evaluation. Option A is nonspecific. Option C and D are common chronic GVHD effects but not alarming for malignancy onset.

SubChapter: Secondary Malignancies – Surveillance

Q495. Answer: C

Explanation: Chronic GVHD prolongs immunosuppression, increasing infection risk; ongoing vaccination and vigilance for symptoms ensure timely management. Option A limits quality of life unnecessarily. Option B endangers safety. Option D lacks evidence and may interfere with medications.

SubChapter: Infection Prevention & Education

Q496. Answer: B

Explanation: Long-term corticosteroid use and chemotherapy contribute to reduced bone mineral density and fracture risk. Option A contributes but is secondary. Option C is unrelated. Option D affects liver and joints, not bone structure directly.

SubChapter: Metabolic Bone Late Effects

Q497. Answer: A

Explanation (50 words): Immunosuppression and chronic GVHD increase skin cancer risk; annual dermatologic examination detects early lesions. Option B aids self-awareness but cannot replace clinical review. Option C delays detection. Option D neglects a known preventable risk.

SubChapter: Secondary Malignancies – Dermatologic

Q498. Answer: B

Explanation: Nurses should promote sleep hygiene, monitor mental health, and collaborate with the medical team; psychological support and medication adjustment may be needed. Option A and D are unsafe without physician oversight. Option C worsens neuropsychiatric effects.

SubChapter: Psychosocial Late Effects

Q499. Answer: B

Explanation: Adequate protein supports tissue repair, while calcium and vitamin D maintain bone health post-steroids. Option A risks iron overload. Option C impairs healing. Option D is unnecessary unless metabolic syndrome exists.

SubChapter: Nutritional Management – Late Recovery

Q500. Answer: B

Explanation: Fertility outcomes vary; reduced-intensity regimens or autologous transplants have higher recovery potential. Option A overstates speed. Option C is incorrect since recovery occurs in some patients. Option D is inaccurate; recovery can occur within two to three years.

SubChapter: Reproductive Health & Counseling

Questions (501-600)

Q501. Late-onset hepatic dysfunction in HSCT survivors is most commonly due to:
A. Hepatitis C infection
B. Chronic GVHD or iron overload
C. Gallstones
D. Biliary atresia

Q502. What education should be emphasized for a patient with ocular GVHD?
A. Use of preservative-free artificial tears
B. Avoid sunglasses
C. Limit fluid intake
D. Stop topical lubricants if symptoms improve

Q503. A 55-year-old HSCT survivor reports persistent fatigue and difficulty concentrating years after recovery. This is most consistent with:
A. Cognitive late effects ("chemo brain")
B. Hypoglycemia
C. Acute infection
D. Thyroid crisis

Q504. Which intervention best supports patient self-management during long-term follow-up?
A. Nurse-led survivorship education and symptom tracking
B. Annual transplant center visits only
C. Medication discontinuation to promote independence
D. Avoid discussing complications

Q505. Late pulmonary fibrosis after HSCT is often linked to:
A. Hypothyroidism
B. CMV infection
C. Hyperbaric oxygen therapy
D. Busulfan-based conditioning regimens

Q506. Which approach promotes best psychosocial recovery in long-term HSCT survivors?
A. Encouraging gradual return to normal roles with counseling support
B. Immediate full workload resumption
C. Avoiding peer groups
D. Ignoring emotional symptoms

Q507. A 44-year-old patient presents two years post-HSCT with progressive shortness of breath and dry cough. Pulmonary function tests show a decline in FEV1. Which late complication is most likely?
A. Chronic obstructive pulmonary disease
B. Bronchiolitis obliterans syndrome
C. Pulmonary embolism
D. Heart failure

Q508. Which late hematologic complication should be screened for annually after allogeneic HSCT?
A. Hemolytic anemia
B. Myelodysplastic syndrome
C. Iron deficiency anemia
D. Polycythemia

Q509. A 60-year-old man with chronic GVHD has persistent oral ulcerations. Which nursing intervention is most appropriate?
A. Alcohol-based mouthwash
B. Frequent saline rinses and topical corticosteroids

C. Avoid all oral rinses
D. High-dose systemic steroids

Q510. What is the primary cause of cataract development in HSCT survivors?
A. Calcineurin inhibitors
B. Total body irradiation
C. Iron overload
D. Dehydration

Q511. A patient six years post-HSCT reports increased fatigue and pallor. Laboratory findings show macrocytosis and low reticulocyte count. Which condition should be suspected?
A. Vitamin B12 deficiency
B. Hemolytic anemia
C. Aplastic relapse
D. Hypersplenism

Q512. Which of the following is most indicative of late chronic GVHD of the liver?
A. Elevated alkaline phosphatase and bilirubin
B. Elevated amylase and lipase
C. Low BUN and creatinine
D. High LDH only

Q513. In long-term HSCT survivors, which infection requires lifelong surveillance due to risk of reactivation?
A. Influenza
B. Cytomegalovirus
C. Hepatitis B
D. Parvovirus B19

Q514. A 45-year-old patient with chronic GVHD complains of dry, thickened skin. Which topical intervention should the nurse recommend?
A. Alcohol-based emollient
B. Lanolin-free moisturizing creams
C. Exfoliating scrubs
D. Corticosteroid patches only

Q515. Which laboratory test best evaluates iron overload in late HSCT survivors?
A. Serum ferritin
B. Total bilirubin
C. Serum calcium
D. C-reactive protein

Q516. A nurse educates a survivor about self-monitoring for chronic GVHD. Which symptom should prompt immediate reporting?
A. Mild appetite loss
B. New joint tightening
C. Occasional fatigue
D. Slight nail changes

Q517. Which lifestyle change most effectively reduces risk for metabolic syndrome post-HSCT?
A. Caloric restriction and regular exercise
B. Avoiding all carbohydrates
C. Increased sodium intake
D. Prolonged rest periods

Q518. A 38-year-old female survivor reports irregular menses and hot flashes two years post-HSCT. Which late effect is suspected?

A. Premature ovarian failure
B. Polycystic ovary syndrome
C. Endometriosis
D. Adrenal insufficiency

Q519. A nurse caring for an HSCT survivor notes persistent hyperglycemia on corticosteroids. What action is most appropriate?

A. Notify provider and reinforce glucose monitoring
B. Stop corticosteroids immediately
C. Double insulin without order
D. Ignore unless symptomatic

Q520. Which patient education point is essential for preventing late infection in splenectomized HSCT survivors?

A. No specific prevention needed
B. Avoid contact with pets
C. Annual pneumococcal and influenza vaccines
D. Routine antiviral prophylaxis only

Q521. Which intervention best supports long-term sexual health after HSCT?

A. Open discussion of intimacy and referral to counseling
B. Avoid sexual activity indefinitely
C. Focus only on fertility, not sexual function
D. Delay discussion until relapse-free for five years

Q522. A patient expresses fear of cancer recurrence years after HSCT. What is the nurse's best response?

A. Provide education on relapse signs and coping resources
B. Minimize concern to reduce anxiety
C. Refer only if physical symptoms appear
D. Avoid discussing psychological issues

Q523. A 47-year-old patient reports brittle nails and hyperpigmented skin patches two years post-HSCT. Which condition should be suspected?

A. Chronic GVHD skin involvement
B. Iron deficiency anemia
C. Fungal infection
D. Autoimmune thyroid disease

Q524. Which teaching point is most important for managing late gastrointestinal complications?

A. Use herbal laxatives regularly
B. Reduce fiber intake
C. Avoid all dairy permanently
D. Report persistent diarrhea or weight loss promptly

Q525. Late pulmonary toxicity is most associated with which chemotherapeutic agent used in conditioning regimens?

A. Busulfan
B. Methotrexate
C. Cyclophosphamide
D. Vincristine

Q526. A long-term survivor experiences difficulty with memory and attention during work tasks. What is the most appropriate nursing action?

A. Recommend cognitive rehabilitation or memory exercises
B. Suggest immediate retirement

C. Increase stimulant medication
D. Ignore symptoms as stress
Q527. A patient presents with chronic diarrhea 18 months post-HSCT and weight loss. Colonoscopy reveals mucosal atrophy and lymphocytic infiltration. What is the most likely diagnosis?
A. Chronic gastrointestinal GVHD
B. CMV colitis
C. Lactose intolerance
D. Bacterial overgrowth
Q528. A 50-year-old survivor develops new shortness of breath and fine bibasilar rales two years after transplant. Chest imaging shows interstitial changes. Which late complication is suspected?
A. Asthma
B. Pleural effusion
C. Pneumocystis pneumonia
D. Pulmonary fibrosis
Q529. A patient complains of jaundice and pruritus three years post-allogeneic transplant. Liver tests reveal elevated alkaline phosphatase and bilirubin. What should the nurse anticipate?
A. Evaluation for chronic hepatic GVHD
B. Vitamin deficiency testing
C. Discontinuation of antivirals
D. Hydration therapy only
Q530. What is the best exercise recommendation for HSCT survivors with long-term fatigue and deconditioning?
A. Gradual aerobic and resistance training
B. High-intensity interval workouts
C. Strict bed rest until energy returns
D. Weightlifting only
Q531. A 55-year-old allogeneic transplant recipient develops thickening of oral mucosa with restricted mouth opening. Which condition is indicated?
A. Sclerotic chronic GVHD
B. Oral candidiasis
C. Xerostomia
D. Aphthous ulceration
Q532. A patient recovering from chronic GVHD asks about long-term immunosuppressive therapy. What should the nurse explain?
A. Alternating agents weekly
B. Stopping immediately after symptoms resolve
C. Using high doses indefinitely
D. Gradual tapering guided by response and infection risk
Q533. What late cardiovascular issue is commonly associated with total body irradiation during conditioning?
A. Accelerated atherosclerosis
B. Pericardial effusion
C. Infective endocarditis
D. Bradyarrhythmia
Q534. A patient reports new wheezing and shortness of breath years after transplant. Pulmonary function testing shows an obstructive pattern unresponsive to bronchodilators. What condition is likely?
A. Bronchiolitis obliterans

B. Asthma
C. Pulmonary embolism
D. Bacterial bronchitis

Q535. A nurse reviews survivorship care with a patient. Which statement indicates correct understanding?

A. "I will maintain yearly visits to monitor late complications."
B. "I can stop all follow-up once I feel healthy."
C. "I don't need to report new skin changes."
D. "Long-term follow-up is only for infections."

Q536. A patient expresses anxiety about resuming employment after prolonged recovery. What is the nurse's best response?

A. Recommend avoiding work indefinitely
B. Advise immediate full-time work
C. Encourage phased return with supportive counseling
D. Focus discussion solely on physical symptoms

Q537. A patient on tacrolimus reports mild tremors and elevated blood pressure. What is the nurse's priority action?

A. Notify provider for possible dose adjustment
B. Discontinue drug immediately
C. Reassure patient it is normal
D. Increase oral fluids only

Q538. In the context of late survivorship, which assessment best evaluates quality of life?

A. Multidimensional fatigue and psychosocial scale
B. Daily temperature log
C. Liver enzyme panel
D. Spirometry alone

Q539. Which teaching topic is essential for HSCT survivors on long-term corticosteroids?

A. Gradual tapering and infection vigilance
B. Abrupt discontinuation when feeling better
C. Doubling dose during fatigue
D. Avoiding all vaccines permanently

Q540. A patient asks how to reduce risk of secondary malignancy after HSCT. Which response is most appropriate?

A. Depend only on immune recovery
B. Use high-dose antioxidants daily
C. Avoid medical follow-ups to limit exposure
D. Maintain cancer screening and sun protection practices

Q541. A 42-year-old survivor presents with chronic cough and mild fever. CT scan shows scattered nodules. Which finding requires immediate consideration?

A. Fungal infection
B. Viral upper respiratory illness
C. Radiation fibrosis
D. Pulmonary edema

Q542. Which nutritional counseling point supports cardiovascular health in long-term HSCT survivors?

A. Emphasize fruits, vegetables, and lean protein intake
B. Increase saturated fat for energy
C. Avoid carbohydrates completely
D. Consume salt freely

Q543. A patient with chronic GVHD skin lesions asks about sun exposure. What should the nurse advise?
A. Limit direct sunlight and use high-SPF sunscreen
B. Increase sun exposure to aid healing
C. Discontinue topical therapy before sun exposure
D. Use tanning beds for vitamin D
Q544. A patient presents five years post-transplant with persistent dyspnea and mild hypoxemia. Which diagnostic study is most useful to evaluate late pulmonary effects?
A. Electrocardiogram
B. Chest X-ray alone
C. High-resolution CT scan
D. Serum ferritin
Q545. What self-care advice supports bone health in HSCT survivors at risk for osteoporosis?
A. Engage in weight-bearing exercise and ensure calcium intake
B. Avoid physical activity
C. Eliminate all dairy products
D. Focus only on vitamin supplements
Q546. A nurse evaluates an HSCT survivor reporting frequent infections years after transplant. Immunoglobulin levels are low. What is the best nursing action?
A. Prepare for possible IV immunoglobulin replacement
B. Encourage herbal immune boosters
C. Recommend discontinuing prophylactic antibiotics
D. Delay further evaluation until next appointment
Q547. A patient reports persistent oral dryness and difficulty swallowing 14 months after HSCT. What nursing intervention is most appropriate?
A. Restrict fluid intake to prevent aspiration
B. Recommend alcohol-based mouthwash
C. Encourage frequent sips of water and saliva substitutes
D. Avoid oral care to reduce irritation
Q548. A 52-year-old allogeneic HSCT survivor develops new-onset hypertension during cyclosporine therapy. What should the nurse anticipate?
A. Medication dose adjustment or switch to tacrolimus
B. Discontinuation of all immunosuppressants
C. Starting over-the-counter diuretics
D. Increasing sodium intake
Q549. A patient two years post-HSCT reports fatigue, pallor, and elevated ferritin. What is the most likely cause?
A. Transfusional iron overload
B. Vitamin B12 deficiency
C. Hypothyroidism
D. Malnutrition
Q550. Which symptom requires urgent evaluation for potential post-transplant lymphoproliferative disorder (PTLD)?
A. Unexplained lymph node enlargement
B. Mild intermittent fever
C. Fatigue relieved by rest
D. Decreased appetite
Q551. What education should be given to a survivor regarding late pulmonary health maintenance?

A. Use antibiotics for every cold
B. Avoid all physical exercise
C. Skip vaccinations if asymptomatic
D. Receive annual influenza and pneumococcal vaccines

Q552. A patient presents with thickened skin, joint stiffness, and reduced range of motion three years post-HSCT. What therapy is most beneficial?

A. Physical therapy with stretching and mobility exercises
B. Extended bed rest
C. Topical antifungals
D. Limiting joint movement

Q553. A patient reports recurrent sinus infections 18 months post-HSCT with low IgG levels. What is the best management approach?

A. Immunoglobulin replacement therapy
B. Oral antihistamines
C. High-dose corticosteroids
D. Decongestant sprays

Q554. Which factor most increases risk for late cataract formation in HSCT survivors?

A. Total body irradiation
B. Chronic dehydration
C. Vitamin A deficiency
D. Hypocalcemia

Q555. A nurse reviews discharge teaching with a patient taking long-term prednisone. Which statement requires further education?

A. "I can stop taking this medication if I feel better."
B. "I'll take it with food to prevent stomach upset."
C. "I should monitor for signs of infection."
D. "I'll report mood changes or weight gain."

Q556. A survivor expresses frustration about persistent fatigue despite remission. What should the nurse emphasize?

A. Fatigue is unrelated to transplant recovery
B. Fatigue means relapse is imminent
C. Bed rest is the best recovery method
D. Fatigue can persist due to long-term treatment effects and needs energy-conservation strategies

Q557. Which intervention best supports late bone health for HSCT survivors on corticosteroids?

A. Calcium and vitamin D supplementation with weight-bearing exercise
B. Reduced protein intake
C. Prolonged immobilization
D. Avoidance of sunlight exposure

Q558. A nurse evaluates a patient two years post-HSCT for late endocrine effects. Which finding warrants further investigation?

A. Fatigue, weight gain, and cold intolerance
B. Mild muscle soreness after exercise
C. Normal energy levels
D. Stable weight and appetite

Q559. Which recommendation promotes effective infection prevention during late recovery?

A. Maintain good hand hygiene and report fever promptly
B. Use antibiotics preemptively
C. Avoid all public places indefinitely

D. Skip dental care appointments

Q560. A 36-year-old patient complains of chronic cough and exertional dyspnea years after transplant. Which late complication is most likely?

A. Pneumonia
B. Asthma
C. Pulmonary embolism
D. Bronchiolitis obliterans

Q561. A nurse teaches a patient about secondary cancer risk reduction. Which statement reflects understanding?

A. "I'll schedule regular skin and oral cancer screenings."
B. "I can skip cancer screenings since my immune system is strong."
C. "Sun exposure helps maintain vitamin D and isn't risky."
D. "I don't need to report new moles."

Q562. Which psychosocial intervention is most effective for anxiety about recurrence?

A. Counseling and support group participation
B. Avoiding discussions of relapse
C. Relying solely on family reassurance
D. Ignoring distress until symptoms worsen

Q563. A patient with chronic GVHD reports severe eye irritation despite lubricating drops. What should the nurse anticipate?

A. Referral for topical cyclosporine therapy
B. Increased use of alcohol-based tears
C. Discontinuing all ocular medications
D. Delaying treatment for six months

Q564. Which long-term complication requires ongoing thyroid function monitoring?

A. Pulmonary edema
B. Renal insufficiency
C. Hepatic steatosis
D. Total body irradiation exposure

Q565. A patient recovering from chronic GVHD is starting to taper immunosuppressive drugs. Which nursing priority is essential?

A. Monitor for early recurrence of skin rash or diarrhea
B. Encourage abrupt discontinuation
C. Decrease follow-up frequency
D. Ignore mild symptoms during taper

Q566. A patient expresses concern about social isolation during long-term recovery. What is the best nursing action?

A. Facilitate support group involvement and gradual social reintegration
B. Advise complete isolation until immune recovery
C. Focus solely on medical aspects of care
D. Suggest family limit emotional discussions

Q567. A 40-year-old HSCT survivor presents with hyperpigmented skin and nail ridging. These findings are most consistent with:

A. Chronic GVHD skin involvement
B. Nutritional deficiency
C. Photosensitivity reaction
D. Fungal infection

Q568. A nurse evaluates a patient two years post-transplant with persistent anemia and elevated ferritin. Which diagnostic test best confirms the suspected complication?
A. Chest X-ray
B. Bone scan
C. Liver MRI for iron quantification
D. Abdominal ultrasound
Q569. A patient reports numbness and tingling in the feet two years after autologous transplant. Which late complication is suspected?
A. Chemotherapy-induced peripheral neuropathy
B. Vitamin K deficiency
C. Autoimmune vasculitis
D. Hypocalcemia
Q570. A 47-year-old survivor asks when it is safe to restart live vaccines. What should the nurse advise?
A. Live vaccines are contraindicated until at least 24 months post-HSCT with confirmed immune recovery
B. They can be resumed six months post-HSCT
C. They are never needed again
D. They can start immediately after engraftment
Q571. A patient complains of shortness of breath and dry cough four years after HSCT. CT scan shows mosaic attenuation and air trapping. What does this indicate?
A. Bronchiolitis obliterans
B. Pulmonary embolism
C. Bacterial pneumonia
D. Pleural effusion
Q572. Which nursing intervention supports sexual health recovery in long-term HSCT survivors?
A. Provide only medication education
B. Advise permanent abstinence
C. Suggest avoiding discussions of sexual function
D. Encourage discussion of intimacy concerns and refer to sexual health counseling
Q573. A patient with chronic GVHD experiences severe skin tightness limiting mobility. What multidisciplinary approach is most effective?
A. Combined physical therapy, topical corticosteroids, and occupational rehabilitation
B. Rest and protective dressings only
C. Increasing systemic steroids alone
D. Avoiding stretching to prevent injury
Q574. A 60-year-old transplant recipient presents with elevated cholesterol and fasting glucose. What should the nurse recommend?
A. Lifestyle modification and metabolic syndrome screening
B. Increased caloric intake
C. Routine steroid escalation
D. Elimination of all carbohydrates
Q575. A patient with chronic GVHD of the liver has pruritus and jaundice. Which medication may help symptom control?
A. Ursodeoxycholic acid
B. Furosemide
C. Prednisone alone
D. Vitamin C supplements

Q576. What nursing teaching supports prevention of secondary skin cancers in HSCT survivors?
A. Skip routine screenings after five years
B. Limit protective clothing to summer months
C. Avoid sunscreen to promote vitamin D
D. Use SPF 30+ sunscreen and schedule annual dermatologic exams
Q577. A patient reports new-onset depression years after HSCT. What is the nurse's most appropriate response?
A. Refer for psychological counseling and assess for support resources
B. Attribute it to normal adjustment
C. Recommend ignoring symptoms
D. Focus solely on physical assessments
Q578. A 35-year-old patient complains of frequent infections despite normal white counts. Immunoglobulin testing shows low IgA. What should the nurse anticipate?
A. IV immunoglobulin replacement and infection precautions
B. No intervention required
C. Broad-spectrum antibiotics indefinitely
D. Discontinuation of vaccinations
Q579. A patient presents with joint pain and stiffness two years after chronic GVHD diagnosis. Which therapy aids long-term mobility?
A. Regular range-of-motion exercises and physical therapy
B. Prolonged immobilization
C. Daily corticosteroid injections
D. Avoiding exercise to prevent pain
Q580. A nurse evaluates a patient experiencing insomnia while on corticosteroids. Which intervention is most helpful?
A. Use sedatives without provider approval
B. Increase caffeine intake during the day
C. Take prednisone at night
D. Encourage morning dosing and relaxation techniques at bedtime
Q581. What education should the nurse provide about alcohol use in HSCT survivors with prior hepatic injury?
A. Avoid alcohol completely to prevent liver damage
B. Moderate intake is safe
C. Alcohol helps appetite recovery
D. Occasional use is inconsequential
Q582. A 57-year-old patient with a history of total body irradiation reports lethargy and weight gain. Which late complication is likely?
A. Hypothyroidism
B. Hyperparathyroidism
C. Adrenal insufficiency
D. Hypoglycemia
Q583. Which preventive strategy helps reduce cardiovascular risk in HSCT survivors?
A. Frequent fasting
B. Avoiding all exercise
C. High-sodium diet
D. Routine lipid monitoring and blood pressure control
Q584. A nurse educates a patient about signs of chronic GVHD recurrence. Which statement indicates understanding?

A. "I'll report any new rash, eye dryness, or mouth soreness immediately."
B. "I'll wait until my next visit to mention symptoms."
C. "Skin dryness is normal and not worth reporting."
D. "GVHD can't return once resolved."

Q585. A 48-year-old survivor complains of decreased concentration and memory lapses. What intervention supports recovery?
A. Cognitive training exercises and structured daily routines
B. Avoid all stimulating activities
C. Increase screen time before bed
D. Depend solely on medication

Q586. Which symptom in a late HSCT survivor warrants immediate evaluation?
A. Unexplained bleeding or bruising
B. Mild fatigue
C. Occasional headache
D. Minor appetite loss

Q587. A survivor reports joint stiffness and thick skin two years post-HSCT. What is the likely cause?
A. Nutrient deficiency
B. Steroid myopathy
C. Viral arthritis
D. Chronic GVHD fibrosis

Q588. A patient with chronic GVHD has persistent dry eyes. What care advice is best?
A. Use artificial tears
B. Avoid sunglasses
C. Reduce fluids
D. Skip eye drops

Q589. A 59-year-old transplant survivor reports cough and exertional dyspnea. CT shows fibrosis. Which agent likely caused this?
A. Busulfan therapy
B. Tacrolimus
C. Methotrexate
D. Filgrastim

Q590. A 42-year-old female reports hot flashes two years post-HSCT. Which effect explains this?
A. Ovarian failure
B. Thyroid disease
C. Diabetes onset
D. Adrenal crisis

Q591. A survivor on steroids has persistent hyperglycemia. What should the nurse do first?
A. Delay action
B. Encourage candy
C. Skip testing
D. Notify provider

Q592. A patient presents with elevated liver enzymes and fatigue. Which late effect is likely?
A. Hepatic GVHD
B. Viral relapse
C. Bone disease
D. Renal injury

Q593. A long-term survivor reports brittle nails and oral dryness. What complication fits best?
A. Chronic GVHD

B. Fungal infection
C. Hypocalcemia
D. Radiation burns

Q594. A 45-year-old survivor with chronic GVHD has persistent rash. What topical treatment helps?

A. Corticosteroid cream
B. Alcohol lotion
C. Antifungal powder
D. Zinc paste

Q595. Which health teaching supports bone protection in HSCT survivors?

A. Low-protein diet
B. Long rest periods
C. Weight-bearing exercise
D. Avoid sunlight

Q596. A 38-year-old man complains of mood changes after prednisone use. What is the best nursing response?

A. Report symptoms
B. Ignore behavior
C. Stop drug
D. Reduce fluids

Q597. A survivor with chronic GVHD skin involvement experiences intense itching. What medication helps relieve this symptom?

A. Antihistamines
B. Diuretics
C. Beta-blockers
D. Antacids

Q598. A patient with chronic GVHD reports difficulty opening the mouth. What therapy promotes improvement?

A. Stretching exercises
B. Ice therapy
C. Oral antibiotics
D. Mouthwash use

Q599. A patient with total body irradiation history reports fatigue and weight gain. What disorder is suspected?

A. Adrenal failure
B. Hyperglycemia
C. Hypocalcemia
D. Hypothyroidism

Q600. A survivor reports blurred vision and light sensitivity. What is the probable cause?

A. Ocular GVHD
B. Iron overload
C. Hypokalemia
D. Diabetes

Answer key and Explanation (501-600)

Q501. Answer: B

Explanation: Chronic GVHD and iron overload are major causes of late hepatic injury post-transplant. Option A occurs rarely now due to donor screening. Option C and D are unrelated to transplant pathology.

SubChapter: Hepatic Late Effects

Q502. Answer: A

Explanation (44 words): Lubrication with preservative-free artificial tears reduces ocular irritation and prevents corneal damage. Option B increases photophobia. Option C is irrelevant. Option D risks symptom recurrence and corneal injury.

SubChapter: Ocular Late Effects – GVHD

Q503. Answer: A

Explanation (47 words): Cognitive impairment from chemotherapy and immunosuppression manifests as memory and attention deficits long-term. Option B produces transient confusion. Option C would include fever or malaise. Option D is acute and life-threatening, not chronic.

SubChapter: Neurocognitive Late Effects

Q504. Answer: A

Explanation (46 words): Structured survivorship programs led by nurses enhance self-monitoring, medication adherence, and early reporting of complications. Option B limits continuity. Option C risks relapse. Option D discourages engagement in care.

SubChapter: Survivorship & Education

Q505. Answer: D

Explanation (45 words): Busulfan and radiation cause interstitial fibrosis due to alveolar injury. Option B can contribute but is less chronic. Option C is therapeutic, not causative. Option A has no pulmonary correlation.

SubChapter: Pulmonary Late Effects – Noninfectious

Q506. Answer: A

Explanation (53 words): Gradual reintegration, supported by counseling and survivorship programs, optimizes emotional and social adjustment. Option B overwhelms patients. Option C removes vital peer support. Option D risks depression and maladaptation.

SubChapter: Psychosocial & Quality-of-Life Management

Q507. Answer: B

Explanation: Bronchiolitis obliterans syndrome is a chronic GVHD-related small airway obstruction common in late survivors. Option A is unrelated unless smoking history exists. Option C causes acute symptoms. Option D produces exertional dyspnea with cardiac findings, not isolated FEV1 decline.

SubChapter: Late Pulmonary Complications

Q508. Answer: B

Explanation: Therapy-related myelodysplastic syndrome can develop years after transplantation due to conditioning-related DNA damage. Option A occurs acutely. Option C is nutritional, not treatment-induced. Option D is unrelated to HSCT.

SubChapter: Hematologic Late Effects

Q509. Answer: B

Explanation: Saline rinses and topical corticosteroids relieve mucosal inflammation without systemic toxicity. Option A irritates tissues. Option C neglects hygiene. Option D is excessive for localized lesions.

SubChapter: Oral Late Effects – GVHD

Q510. Answer: B

Explanation: Total body irradiation damages lens proteins, leading to opacification years later. Option A affects kidneys. Option C causes hepatic, not ocular issues. Option D has no ocular impact.

SubChapter: Ocular Late Effects – Radiation

Q511. Answer: A

Explanation: Vitamin B12 deficiency is a recognized late nutritional effect after prolonged immunosuppression and altered absorption. Option B shows elevated reticulocytes. Option C presents with pancytopenia. Option D would cause sequestration, not macrocytosis.

SubChapter: Nutritional & Hematologic Late Effects

Q512. Answer: A

Explanation: Liver involvement in chronic GVHD shows cholestatic patterns with raised alkaline phosphatase and bilirubin. Option B suggests pancreatitis. Option C reflects renal function. Option D alone lacks specificity.

SubChapter: Hepatic Late Effects – Chronic GVHD

Q513. Answer: B

Explanation: CMV can reactivate in immunocompromised states even years post-transplant. Option A requires annual vaccination. Option C persists but is managed with antiviral prophylaxis in known carriers. Option D rarely causes chronic infection.

SubChapter: Late Infectious Complications

Q514. Answer: B

Explanation: Lanolin-free emollients preserve moisture and reduce irritation in sclerodermatous GVHD. Option A worsens dryness. Option C causes microtrauma. Option D may help localized lesions but not global care.

SubChapter: Dermatologic Late Effects

Q515. Answer: A

Explanation: Ferritin is the preferred screening biomarker for transfusional iron overload in long-term follow-up. Option B indicates liver function. Option C and D measure unrelated parameters.

SubChapter: Metabolic Late Effects

Q516. Answer: B

Explanation: New contractures or stiffness may signal sclerotic GVHD progression needing early treatment. Options A, C, and D are minor unless persistent or worsening.

SubChapter: Patient Education – Chronic GVHD

Q517. Answer: A

Explanation: Balanced diet and exercise control weight, glucose, and lipid profiles altered by immunosuppressive therapy. Option B is extreme. Option C elevates blood pressure. Option D worsens deconditioning.

SubChapter: Health Promotion – Metabolic

Q518. Answer: A

Explanation: Alkylating agents and total body irradiation can cause ovarian failure leading to menopausal symptoms. Option B causes irregular menses but not vasomotor symptoms. Option C is unrelated. Option D presents with fatigue and hypotension.

SubChapter: Endocrine & Reproductive Late Effects

Q519. Answer: A

Explanation: Collaboration ensures proper adjustment and early detection of steroid-induced diabetes. Option B risks GVHD flare. Option C exceeds nursing scope. Option D delays management.

SubChapter: Metabolic Late Effects – Corticosteroid-Related

Q520. Answer: C

Explanation: Loss of splenic function increases susceptibility to encapsulated bacteria, making vaccination crucial. Option B is unnecessary. Option A ignores infection risk. Option D does not cover bacterial pathogens.

SubChapter: Infection Prevention – Functional Asplenia

Q521. Answer: A
Explanation: Early, open dialogue normalizes sexual health concerns and facilitates recovery. Option B fosters anxiety. Option C omits psychosocial needs. Option D delays essential support.
SubChapter: Sexual Health & Psychosocial Support
Q522. Answer: A
Explanation: Honest education and emotional support empower patients, improving self-efficacy. Option B invalidates feelings. Option C delays help. Option D neglects mental health.
SubChapter: Psychosocial Care – Fear of Recurrence
Q523. Answer: A
Explanation: Skin and nail changes often reflect chronic GVHD with immune-mediated epithelial injury. Option B causes pallor, not pigmentation. Option C produces localized lesions. Option D affects metabolism, not nails.
SubChapter: Dermatologic Late Effects
Q524. Answer: D
Explanation: Persistent diarrhea may signal GVHD or malabsorption; prompt evaluation prevents dehydration and nutrient loss. Option B may worsen constipation. Option C is unnecessary unless intolerant. Option A is unsafe chronically.
SubChapter: Gastrointestinal Late Effects
Q525. Answer: A
Explanation: Busulfan induces dose-dependent pulmonary fibrosis as a late complication. Option B affects liver and mucosa. Option C causes cystitis. Option D is neurotoxic, not pulmonary.
SubChapter: Pulmonary Late Effects – Chemotherapy-Related
Q526. Answer: A
Explanation: Cognitive rehabilitation and structured memory strategies help manage post-treatment cognitive dysfunction ("chemo brain"). Option B reduces self-esteem. Option C requires medical supervision. Option D dismisses valid symptoms.
SubChapter: Neurocognitive & Educational Support
Q527. Answer: A
Explanation: Chronic gastrointestinal GVHD leads to immune-mediated mucosal damage, resulting in malabsorption and persistent diarrhea. CMV colitis presents acutely with ulcerations, lactose intolerance lacks inflammation, and bacterial overgrowth responds rapidly to antibiotics rather than immunosuppressive therapy.
SubChapter: Gastrointestinal Late Effects – Chronic GVHD
Q528. Answer: D
Explanation: Pulmonary fibrosis results from previous chemotherapy, total body irradiation, or chronic GVHD and manifests as restrictive interstitial disease. Pleural effusion causes fluid accumulation, pneumocystis is acute and infectious, and asthma produces reversible airway obstruction rather than fibrotic patterns.
SubChapter: Pulmonary Late Effects – Fibrotic
Q529. Answer: A
Explanation: Chronic hepatic GVHD causes cholestatic jaundice due to bile duct inflammation and fibrosis. Vitamin deficiency does not elevate cholestatic enzymes, antiviral withdrawal could worsen viral reactivation, and hydration alone does not correct immune-mediated liver injury.
SubChapter: Hepatic Late Effects – GVHD
Q530. Answer: A
Explanation: Structured, progressive aerobic and resistance exercise improves stamina, muscle strength, and psychosocial wellbeing. High-intensity regimens risk exhaustion, bed rest worsens weakness, and single-modality weightlifting neglects cardiovascular endurance essential for recovery.

SubChapter: Physical Rehabilitation & Fatigue

Q531. Answer: A

Explanation: Sclerotic chronic GVHD causes fibrotic mucosal contraction limiting oral opening. Candidiasis appears with white plaques, xerostomia involves dryness without fibrosis, and aphthous ulcers are isolated painful lesions not associated with sclerosis.

SubChapter: Oral Late Effects – GVHD

Q532. Answer: D

Explanation: Immunosuppressants require individualized tapering to balance GVHD control and infection prevention. Abrupt cessation risks relapse, indefinite high dosing increases toxicity, and alternating regimens weekly provides no stability in immune suppression or monitoring.

SubChapter: Pharmacologic Management – Immunosuppression

Q533. Answer: A

Explanation: Radiation exposure accelerates endothelial injury leading to premature atherosclerosis and coronary artery disease. Pericardial effusion arises acutely from inflammation, endocarditis is infectious, and bradyarrhythmia is unrelated to irradiation dose.

SubChapter: Cardiovascular Late Effects

Q534. Answer: A

Explanation: Bronchiolitis obliterans is a chronic nonreversible airway obstruction due to immune injury, common in late survivors. Asthma typically improves with bronchodilators, embolism presents abruptly, and bacterial bronchitis resolves with antibiotics.

SubChapter: Pulmonary Late Effects – Chronic GVHD

Q535. Answer: A

Explanation: Lifelong follow-up enables early detection of chronic GVHD, endocrine changes, and secondary malignancies. Ending follow-up prematurely or ignoring dermatologic signs increases morbidity, and surveillance includes multiple organ systems beyond infection control.

SubChapter: Survivorship & Education

Q536. Answer: C

Explanation: A gradual, supported return promotes adaptation and confidence, while addressing both physical and psychosocial needs. Immediate full-time workload risks exhaustion, permanent avoidance hinders recovery, and ignoring emotional concerns neglects holistic care.

SubChapter: Psychosocial & Occupational Reintegration

Q537. Answer: A

Explanation: Tacrolimus toxicity manifests as tremors and hypertension requiring prompt evaluation and potential dose change. Abrupt discontinuation can trigger GVHD, reassurance alone ignores potential harm, and hydration does not mitigate neurotoxic effects.

SubChapter: Medication Monitoring – Immunosuppressants

Q538. Answer: A

Explanation: Multidimensional scales assess emotional, physical, and social wellbeing, offering a comprehensive quality-of-life view. Temperature logs detect infection only, liver tests and spirometry address organ-specific issues but not holistic function or adjustment.

SubChapter: Quality of Life & Assessment

Q539. Answer: A

Explanation: Gradual tapering prevents adrenal insufficiency, and monitoring for infection addresses immune suppression risks. Sudden cessation may cause adrenal crisis, increasing doses independently is unsafe, and vaccination schedules resume as immune function returns.

SubChapter: Pharmacologic Late Effects – Corticosteroids

Q540. Answer: D

Explanation: Regular screenings and sun safety significantly lower secondary cancer risk. High-dose supplements lack evidence, avoiding checkups delays detection, and relying solely on immune restoration neglects environmental and treatment-related risks.
SubChapter: Secondary Malignancies – Prevention

Q541. Answer: A

Explanation: Immunosuppressed HSCT patients are prone to opportunistic fungal infections that can present insidiously with nodules. Viral infections are self-limited, radiation fibrosis lacks fever, and edema causes diffuse infiltrates rather than nodular lesions.
SubChapter: Late Infectious Complications

Q542. Answer: A

Explanation: A balanced diet rich in plant foods and lean proteins helps control cholesterol and reduce radiation-induced vascular risk. High-fat or high-salt diets promote atherosclerosis, while carbohydrate elimination leads to nutrient imbalance.
SubChapter: Nutritional Management – Cardiovascular Health

Q543. Answer: A

Explanation: Photosensitivity and malignancy risk are heightened by immunosuppressants and GVHD, making sun avoidance and protection critical. Excessive exposure worsens lesions, stopping topical care is counterproductive, and tanning increases cancer risk.
SubChapter: Skin Care & Safety Education

Q544. Answer: C

Explanation: High-resolution CT provides detailed imaging to identify fibrosis or bronchiolitis obliterans characteristic of late pulmonary complications. Standard radiographs may miss subtle changes, ECG evaluates cardiac issues, and ferritin reflects iron overload unrelated to lung pathology.
SubChapter: Diagnostic Evaluation – Pulmonary

Q545. Answer: A

Explanation: Weight-bearing activity and adequate calcium enhance bone strength and counteract steroid-induced osteoporosis. Sedentary behavior accelerates bone loss, dairy avoidance reduces calcium intake, and supplements alone cannot replace mechanical bone stimulation.
SubChapter: Musculoskeletal Late Effects

Q546. Answer: A

Explanation: Persistent hypogammaglobulinemia requires IV immunoglobulin therapy to restore immune protection and prevent severe infections. Herbal supplements lack evidence, stopping prophylaxis increases risk, and deferring evaluation may endanger patient safety.
SubChapter: Immune Reconstitution & Infection Prevention

Q547. Answer: C

Explanation: Chronic GVHD frequently causes xerostomia; hydration and saliva substitutes relieve symptoms and maintain mucosal health. Alcohol-based rinses exacerbate dryness, fluid restriction increases discomfort, and neglecting oral care promotes mucosal injury and infection.
SubChapter: Oral Late Effects – Chronic GVHD

Q548. Answer: A

Explanation: Cyclosporine-induced vasoconstriction commonly elevates blood pressure, requiring dose modification or alternative immunosuppressive therapy. Abrupt cessation risks GVHD, unsupervised diuretics are unsafe, and increased sodium worsens hypertension.
SubChapter: Cardiovascular & Renal Late Effects

Q549. Answer: A

Explanation: Multiple transfusions during and after transplant lead to iron accumulation, resulting in fatigue, hepatic dysfunction, and elevated ferritin. Vitamin deficiency or thyroid issues cause anemia without iron excess, and malnutrition produces broader deficiencies rather than ferritin elevation.

SubChapter: Metabolic Late Effects – Iron Overload

Q550. Answer: A

Explanation: Persistent or rapidly enlarging lymph nodes may indicate PTLD, a potentially fatal Epstein-Barr virus–driven complication. Low-grade fever, fatigue, and appetite loss are nonspecific and typically accompany benign post-treatment effects rather than malignancy.

SubChapter: Secondary Malignancies – PTLD

Q551. Answer: D

Explanation: Annual vaccination prevents respiratory infections that can worsen underlying pulmonary compromise. Avoiding activity leads to deconditioning, neglecting vaccines invites preventable illness, and unnecessary antibiotics contribute to resistance without addressing viral pathogens.

SubChapter: Infection Prevention – Pulmonary

Q552. Answer: A

Explanation: Regular physical therapy minimizes contractures and maintains flexibility in sclerotic chronic GVHD. Immobility accelerates fibrosis, antifungals are irrelevant, and limiting movement worsens functional decline.

SubChapter: Musculoskeletal Late Effects – GVHD

Q553. Answer: A

Explanation: Hypogammaglobulinemia predisposes patients to recurrent bacterial infections; IV or subcutaneous immunoglobulin restores antibody levels and prevents severe illness. Symptomatic agents do not address the underlying immune deficiency.

SubChapter: Immune Reconstitution – Hypogammaglobulinemia

Q554. Answer: A

Explanation: Total body irradiation damages lens proteins, leading to cataract development years later. Dehydration and mineral or vitamin imbalances do not cause this structural ocular change.

SubChapter: Ocular Late Effects – Radiation

Q555. Answer: A

Explanation: Prednisone must be tapered gradually under medical supervision to prevent adrenal crisis. Taking it with food reduces gastric irritation, infection monitoring ensures safety, and reporting emotional or physical changes allows timely intervention.

SubChapter: Pharmacologic Management – Corticosteroids

Q556. Answer: D

Explanation: Post-transplant fatigue is multifactorial, influenced by anemia, hormonal imbalance, and deconditioning. Structured activity and rest balance promote improvement, while catastrophic or dismissive explanations hinder adaptation and emotional health.

SubChapter: Psychosocial & Physical Rehabilitation

Q557. Answer: A

Explanation: Adequate calcium, vitamin D, and regular weight-bearing activity prevent steroid-induced osteoporosis. Low-protein diets impair bone repair, immobility accelerates demineralization, and total sun avoidance limits natural vitamin D synthesis.

SubChapter: Musculoskeletal Late Effects – Osteoporosis

Q558. Answer: A

Explanation: Hypothyroidism is a common late effect, presenting with fatigue, weight gain, and cold intolerance. Other listed conditions are within expected recovery variations and do not indicate endocrine dysfunction.

SubChapter: Endocrine Late Effects – Thyroid

Q559. Answer: A

Explanation: Hand hygiene and early symptom reporting are central to infection prevention. Unnecessary antibiotic use promotes resistance, prolonged isolation harms mental health, and poor dental care increases bacterial risk.
SubChapter: Infection Prevention – Education

Q560. Answer: D

Explanation: Bronchiolitis obliterans causes progressive airflow obstruction secondary to chronic GVHD or chemotherapy toxicity. Asthma typically reverses with bronchodilators, embolism presents acutely, and pneumonia produces fever and infiltrates rather than persistent airflow limitation.
SubChapter: Pulmonary Late Effects – Chronic GVHD

Q561. Answer: A

Explanation: Routine screenings allow early detection of radiation- or drug-related malignancies. Avoiding surveillance or ignoring skin changes increases risk, and excessive sun exposure is a recognized carcinogenic factor.
SubChapter: Secondary Malignancies – Surveillance

Q562. Answer: A

Explanation: Structured counseling and peer groups normalize experiences and provide coping strategies, reducing anxiety and isolation. Avoidance or denial limits adjustment, and dependence solely on family lacks therapeutic guidance.
SubChapter: Psychosocial Support – Fear of Recurrence

Q563. Answer: A

Explanation: Topical cyclosporine reduces inflammation and improves tear production in refractory ocular GVHD. Alcohol-based tears worsen irritation, cessation of therapy risks damage, and delaying treatment allows progression to corneal injury.
SubChapter: Ocular Late Effects – GVHD

Q564. Answer: D

Explanation: Total body irradiation damages thyroid tissue, causing delayed hypothyroidism that necessitates regular hormonal screening. Renal, hepatic, or pulmonary disorders do not directly impair thyroid regulation.
SubChapter: Endocrine Late Effects – Radiation

Q565. Answer: A

Explanation: Recurrence of GVHD often appears first as rash or diarrhea during tapering, requiring prompt evaluation. Abrupt cessation heightens relapse risk, less monitoring delays response, and ignoring early warning signs leads to severe complications.
SubChapter: Immunosuppression Management – GVHD Monitoring

Q566. Answer: A

Explanation: Structured social engagement and peer support enhance emotional resilience and reintegration. Prolonged isolation harms psychological wellbeing, exclusive focus on medical aspects ignores holistic care, and discouraging communication weakens coping capacity.
SubChapter: Psychosocial Rehabilitation & Education

Q567. Answer: A

Explanation: Chronic GVHD often produces pigmentation changes and nail dystrophy from immune-mediated epithelial damage. Nutritional deficiency causes brittle nails but not pigmentation, photosensitivity presents with erythema, and fungal infection results in localized discoloration rather than systemic nail changes.
SubChapter: Dermatologic Late Effects – Chronic GVHD

Q568. Answer: C

Explanation: Liver MRI accurately measures hepatic iron concentration and confirms transfusional iron overload, a frequent late effect. Bone scans detect skeletal metastases, chest X-rays assess pulmonary issues, and ultrasound cannot quantify iron burden precisely.
SubChapter: Metabolic Late Effects – Iron Overload

Q569. Answer: A

Explanation: Agents like vincristine and cisplatin cause long-lasting peripheral neuropathy due to neuronal injury. Vitamin K and calcium abnormalities do not cause sensory loss, and vasculitis presents with pain and inflammation rather than chronic numbness.
SubChapter: Neurologic Late Effects – Chemotherapy

Q570. Answer: A

Explanation: Live vaccines are safe only once immune reconstitution is documented, typically after two years, to prevent vaccine-related infection. Early administration risks disease, while skipping vaccination leaves the patient unprotected.
SubChapter: Immune Reconstitution & Vaccination

Q571. Answer: A

Explanation: Mosaic attenuation and air trapping are radiologic hallmarks of bronchiolitis obliterans, a late noninfectious complication of chronic GVHD. Embolism and effusion produce localized findings, while pneumonia shows consolidation, not airway obstruction.
SubChapter: Pulmonary Late Effects – Chronic GVHD

Q572. Answer: D

Explanation: Open communication normalizes sexual health topics and facilitates counseling for hormonal or psychological issues. Avoidance or abstinence worsens isolation, and limiting education to medications overlooks emotional and relational aspects.
SubChapter: Psychosocial & Reproductive Health

Q573. Answer: A

Explanation: Integrated therapy addresses inflammation, fibrosis, and mobility simultaneously, improving quality of life. Rest alone fosters contractures, high-dose steroids cause toxicity without full relief, and lack of stretching worsens stiffness.
SubChapter: Musculoskeletal Late Effects – GVHD

Q574. Answer: A

Explanation: Metabolic syndrome is a common late complication from corticosteroid use and inactivity; early lifestyle intervention and monitoring prevent cardiovascular disease. Excess calories or extreme dietary restriction worsen health risks.
SubChapter: Metabolic Late Effects – Cardiovascular

Q575. Answer: A

Explanation: Ursodeoxycholic acid improves bile flow and reduces pruritus in cholestatic liver GVHD. Diuretics treat edema, corticosteroids reduce inflammation but not bile flow, and vitamin supplements have no effect on hepatic cholestasis.
SubChapter: Hepatic Late Effects – GVHD

Q576. Answer: D

Explanation: Sun protection and regular skin exams detect early malignancies related to immunosuppression and radiation. Neglecting sunscreen or screenings increases risk, and seasonal protection alone fails to prevent year-round UV exposure.
SubChapter: Secondary Malignancies – Skin

Q577. Answer: A

Explanation: Psychological counseling and support referrals address long-term emotional impacts of transplant, improving adherence and quality of life. Minimizing symptoms delays recovery, and exclusive physical focus overlooks mental health needs.

SubChapter: Psychosocial Late Effects – Depression
Q578. Answer: A
Explanation: Persistent IgA deficiency compromises mucosal immunity, requiring immunoglobulin therapy and preventive education. Ignoring the issue risks recurrent infection, continuous antibiotics promote resistance, and stopping vaccines removes protection against other pathogens.
SubChapter: Immune Reconstitution – Deficiency
Q579. Answer: A
Explanation: Exercise preserves flexibility and counters fibrosis in sclerotic GVHD. Immobility leads to contractures, repeated steroid injections raise infection risk, and avoiding activity worsens stiffness and discomfort.
SubChapter: Musculoskeletal Rehabilitation – GVHD
Q580. Answer: D
Explanation: Administering steroids in the morning aligns with circadian rhythm, reducing insomnia, while relaxation strategies improve sleep hygiene. Caffeine or nighttime dosing worsens symptoms, and unsupervised sedative use poses safety risks.
SubChapter: Pharmacologic Late Effects – Corticosteroids
Q581. Answer: A
Explanation: Alcohol increases hepatotoxicity risk in patients with prior hepatic injury or GVHD. Abstinence preserves liver health; even small amounts may compound damage caused by previous conditioning and immunosuppressants.
SubChapter: Hepatic Late Effects – Education
Q582. Answer: A
Explanation: Radiation-induced thyroid injury leads to decreased hormone production, causing lethargy and weight gain. Parathyroid disorders affect calcium levels, adrenal issues present with hypotension, and hypoglycemia produces episodic weakness, not chronic fatigue.
SubChapter: Endocrine Late Effects – Thyroid
Q583. Answer: D
Explanation: Regular monitoring and risk factor management mitigate late vascular toxicity from conditioning and immunosuppressants. Sedentary lifestyle, excess sodium, and extreme fasting elevate cardiovascular strain and metabolic imbalance.
SubChapter: Cardiovascular Health – Prevention
Q584. Answer: A
Explanation: Early recognition and reporting of recurrence signs enable prompt treatment and prevent severe organ involvement. Delaying notification or dismissing symptoms risks irreversible complications, and assuming permanent resolution ignores relapse potential.
SubChapter: Education & Self-Management – GVHD
Q585. Answer: A
Explanation: Cognitive rehabilitation enhances attention and executive function impaired by chemotherapy or irradiation. Overstimulation and medication dependence hinder adaptation, while structured tasks promote mental retraining and confidence.
SubChapter: Neurocognitive Rehabilitation
Q586. Answer: A
Explanation: Spontaneous bleeding may signal thrombocytopenia or secondary marrow failure requiring urgent assessment. Mild fatigue and appetite changes are common recovery issues and not immediately life-threatening without additional signs.
SubChapter: Hematologic Late Effects – Surveillance
Q587. Answer: D

Explanation: Chronic GVHD triggers fibrotic tissue remodeling, producing skin tightness and restricted mobility. Steroid myopathy weakens muscles without sclerosis, viral arthritis causes transient inflammation, and nutrient deficits do not create contractures or dermal thickening.
SubChapter: Musculoskeletal Late Effects – GVHD

Q588. Answer: A

Explanation: Artificial tears relieve dryness, protect the cornea, and maintain comfort in ocular GVHD. Sun avoidance and hydration are important, but stopping drops or reducing fluids worsens irritation and ocular surface damage.
SubChapter: Ocular Late Effects – GVHD

Q589. Answer: A

Explanation: Busulfan leads to dose-dependent pulmonary fibrosis through alveolar damage and oxidative stress. Tacrolimus affects kidneys, methotrexate causes hepatic toxicity, and filgrastim stimulates marrow without lung injury.
SubChapter: Pulmonary Late Effects – Chemotherapy

Q590. Answer: A

Explanation: Alkylating agents and radiation can destroy ovarian tissue, leading to premature menopause with vasomotor symptoms. Thyroid and adrenal disorders cause metabolic changes, not flushing or cycle loss, and diabetes produces thirst and fatigue.
SubChapter: Endocrine Late Effects – Reproductive

Q591. Answer: D

Explanation: Corticosteroids elevate glucose through insulin resistance; notifying the provider enables timely dose or therapy adjustment. Excess sugar worsens levels, ignoring tests hides complications, and delay risks metabolic crisis.
SubChapter: Metabolic Late Effects – Corticosteroids

Q592. Answer: A

Explanation: Immune-mediated bile duct inflammation in hepatic GVHD elevates transaminases and causes malaise. Viral relapse is less chronic, bone and renal diseases produce unrelated laboratory changes.
SubChapter: Hepatic Late Effects – GVHD

Q593. Answer: A

Explanation: GVHD affects epithelial cells, leading to dry mucosa and fragile nails from autoimmune damage. Fungal infections are localized, calcium deficiency affects muscle tone, and radiation burns occur acutely, not years later.
SubChapter: Dermatologic Late Effects – GVHD

Q594. Answer: A

Explanation: Topical corticosteroids reduce localized inflammation and immune infiltration characteristic of GVHD rash. Alcohol irritates skin, antifungal agents treat infections, and zinc paste soothes irritation without addressing immune etiology.
SubChapter: Dermatologic Late Effects – Treatment

Q595. Answer: C

Explanation: Regular exercise maintains bone density and prevents steroid-induced osteoporosis. Prolonged rest accelerates demineralization, reduced protein limits bone repair, and avoiding sunlight restricts vitamin D synthesis needed for calcium absorption.
SubChapter: Musculoskeletal Late Effects – Osteoporosis

Q596. Answer: A

Explanation: Corticosteroids can cause mood swings or irritability; timely reporting allows safe evaluation and medication adjustment. Ignoring signs or abrupt withdrawal is unsafe, and hydration has no therapeutic impact.

SubChapter: Psychosocial & Pharmacologic Late Effects

Q597. Answer: A

Explanation: Antihistamines alleviate pruritus by blocking histamine receptors and providing comfort. Diuretics address fluid overload, beta-blockers manage hypertension, and antacids target gastric issues unrelated to skin symptoms.

SubChapter: Dermatologic Late Effects – Symptom Control

Q598. Answer: A

Explanation: Regular stretching maintains oral mobility and prevents fibrosis progression in sclerotic GVHD. Ice therapy offers short-term relief, antibiotics are for infection, and mouthwash does not restore range of motion.

SubChapter: Oral Late Effects – Rehabilitation

Q599. Answer: D

Explanation: Radiation impairs thyroid tissue, leading to reduced hormone output, fatigue, and metabolic slowing. High glucose levels cause thirst and polyuria, calcium and adrenal abnormalities display different systemic effects.

SubChapter: Endocrine Late Effects – Thyroid

Q600. Answer: A

Explanation: Ocular GVHD produces dryness and photophobia due to lacrimal gland inflammation. Iron overload affects liver, potassium imbalance causes muscle issues, and diabetes-related retinopathy develops more gradually with different patterns.

SubChapter: Ocular Late Effects – GVHD

Questions (601-700)

Q601. Which lifestyle guidance benefits cardiovascular health after HSCT?

A. Balanced diet and walking
B. High-fat meals
C. Smoking resumption
D. Irregular exercise

Q602. A survivor experiences new oral ulcerations with burning pain. What condition should be assessed?

A. Iron deficiency
B. Fungal thrush
C. Mucosal GVHD
D. Allergy reaction

Q603. A 50-year-old patient notes easy bruising and petechiae years post-HSCT. Which condition is most concerning?

A. Secondary marrow failure
B. Vitamin deficiency
C. Allergy rash
D. Mild dehydration

Q604. Which teaching point supports immune recovery education?

A. Maintain hygiene and avoid live vaccines
B. Skip all boosters
C. Avoid routine follow-up
D. Discontinue prophylaxis

Q605. A survivor reports tingling fingers after long-term tacrolimus use. What side effect is likely?

A. Neurotoxicity
B. Hypocalcemia
C. Fatigue
D. Myalgia

Q606. A 47-year-old survivor states, "I'm afraid the cancer will return." What should the nurse do?

A. Avoid topic
B. Dismiss fear
C. Offer counseling referral
D. Delay support

Q607. A 39-year-old survivor complains of progressive shortness of breath and wheezing unresponsive to inhalers. Spirometry shows an obstructive pattern. What is the likely cause?

A. Bronchiolitis obliterans
B. Asthma
C. Pulmonary edema
D. Pneumonia

Q608. A 55-year-old male survivor has elevated cholesterol and mild hypertension. What nursing teaching is most appropriate?

A. Adopt low-fat diet and regular exercise
B. Restrict fluids and protein intake
C. Increase sodium for hydration
D. Avoid all physical activity

Q609. A patient two years post-HSCT reports persistent cough and dyspnea on exertion. HRCT reveals interstitial infiltrates. Which cause is most likely?

A. Pulmonary fibrosis
B. Acute infection
C. Fluid overload
D. Embolism

Q610. A survivor expresses guilt for depending on family during recovery. What nursing intervention is best?
A. Focus only on medication adherence
B. Avoid discussing emotions
C. Suggest isolation for reflection
D. Encourage counseling and gradual role resumption

Q611. A 50-year-old patient treated with total body irradiation reports cold intolerance and weight gain. Which complication should the nurse suspect?
A. Hypothyroidism
B. Diabetes mellitus
C. Adrenal insufficiency
D. Hypoglycemia

Q612. A 46-year-old allogeneic transplant survivor has new right upper quadrant pain and pruritus. Labs show high alkaline phosphatase. What should be suspected?
A. Hepatic chronic GVHD
B. Viral hepatitis
C. Renal failure
D. Gallstones

Q613. A patient with chronic GVHD reports eye pain and excessive tearing. What is the most appropriate nursing action?
A. Refer to ophthalmology for cyclosporine drops
B. Recommend over-the-counter redness drops
C. Reduce fluid intake
D. Avoid all eye medications

Q614. A survivor on prednisone reports difficulty sleeping and irritability. What advice should the nurse provide?
A. Skip doses to rest better
B. Take the dose at night before bed
C. Take medication in the morning and maintain a bedtime routine
D. Increase caffeine to stay alert

Q615. A 60-year-old HSCT survivor reports fatigue and darkening skin. Ferritin levels are markedly elevated. What is the appropriate management step?
A. Initiate iron chelation therapy
B. Begin vitamin B12 supplements
C. Reduce dietary protein
D. Encourage more rest

Q616. A patient experiencing chronic GVHD skin sclerosis asks how to maintain mobility. What should the nurse suggest?
A. Daily stretching and physical therapy
B. Frequent rest and immobilization
C. Cold compresses alone
D. Massage without exercise

Q617. A 35-year-old woman experiences infertility two years after myeloablative conditioning. What explanation should be provided?

A. Ovarian failure from chemotherapy and radiation
B. Temporary suppression from medications
C. Stress-induced cycle change
D. Infection-related scarring

Q618. A 58-year-old survivor on tacrolimus reports hand tremors and mild hypertension. What does this indicate?

A. Calcium loss
B. Adrenal crisis
C. Anxiety disorder
D. Drug toxicity

Q619. A survivor describes emotional numbness and fear of future illness. What nursing intervention supports recovery?

A. Facilitate referral to mental health and survivorship programs
B. Recommend solitary reflection without therapy
C. Emphasize only physical strength training
D. Delay discussion until next visit

Q620. A patient reports recurrent sinus infections and low immunoglobulin levels 18 months post-transplant. What should the nurse anticipate?

A. IV immunoglobulin replacement
B. Broad antibiotic prophylaxis
C. Daily antihistamine therapy
D. Nasal steroid spray

Q621. A 48-year-old patient reports sudden joint swelling and skin tightness. Which intervention is most important?

A. Prompt evaluation for sclerotic GVHD
B. Apply topical antifungal cream
C. Encourage rest without movement
D. Begin physical therapy independently

Q622. A survivor complains of chronic dry mouth, altered taste, and poor appetite. What management is appropriate?

A. Skip dental checkups
B. Avoid fluids during meals
C. Increase salt intake
D. Use saliva substitutes and frequent oral care

Q623. A patient's family expresses concern about memory loss and reduced focus years after HSCT. What support should the nurse recommend?

A. Cognitive therapy and mental exercises
B. Sedative use for rest
C. Ignore mild forgetfulness
D. Isolate from stimuli

Q624. A 45-year-old HSCT survivor reports persistent cough and fever. Imaging shows multiple nodules. What is the nurse's concern?

A. Fungal pneumonia
B. Viral bronchitis
C. Radiation pneumonitis
D. Pulmonary embolism

Q625. A patient on long-term corticosteroids reports vision changes. Which late effect is suspected?

A. Cataract formation

B. Retinal detachment
C. Optic neuritis
D. Glaucoma

Q626. A survivor with chronic GVHD skin lesions asks about safe outdoor activities. What education is most important?

A. Sun exposure helps improve lesions
B. Use sunscreen, protective clothing, and limit direct sun
C. Stop medications before outdoor activity
D. Avoid outdoor activity completely

Q627. A 49-year-old survivor presents with progressive cough and shortness of breath 18 months post-HSCT. HRCT reveals small airway narrowing. What is the diagnosis?

A. Bronchiolitis obliterans
B. Pleural effusion
C. Pulmonary embolism
D. Asthma

Q628. A survivor reports persistent dry, painful mouth with sensitivity to spicy food. What care measure should be emphasized?

A. Use bland rinses and saliva substitutes regularly
B. Rinse with alcohol mouthwash after meals
C. Eat acidic foods to stimulate saliva
D. Reduce oral hygiene frequency

Q629. A 53-year-old HSCT survivor experiences bone pain and multiple vertebral fractures. What complication should the nurse suspect?

A. Steroid-induced osteoporosis
B. Calcium deficiency
C. Vitamin A toxicity
D. Iron overload

Q630. A 41-year-old female survivor reports irregular menses and infertility after myeloablative conditioning. Which hormone is most likely deficient?

A. Aldosterone
B. Cortisol
C. Insulin
D. Estrogen

Q631. A patient with chronic GVHD develops yellow sclera and pruritus. Labs show elevated bilirubin and alkaline phosphatase. What treatment may help?

A. Ursodeoxycholic acid
B. Antifungal therapy
C. High-protein diet
D. Iron supplements

Q632. A 57-year-old survivor experiences forgetfulness and difficulty multitasking. What intervention should be prioritized?

A. Cognitive rehabilitation program
B. Sedative at bedtime
C. Vitamin C supplementation
D. Reduced social activity

Q633. A 45-year-old patient reports chronic fatigue and mild depression during long-term follow-up. Which recommendation supports recovery?

A. Regular light exercise and counseling support

B. Avoid physical activity and rest excessively
C. Rely solely on medication for energy
D. Ignore emotional distress

Q634. A patient reports thickened skin and reduced finger flexibility. What should the nurse recommend?

A. Avoiding physical therapy
B. Limiting hand movement
C. Applying alcohol gel frequently
D. Daily stretching and moisturizing

Q635. A 62-year-old HSCT survivor develops blurred vision and glare sensitivity. Which complication is likely?

A. Cataract formation
B. Optic neuritis
C. Retinal detachment
D. Conjunctivitis

Q636. A patient's partner reports the survivor has become socially withdrawn after recovery. What is the nurse's best intervention?

A. Facilitate mental health referral and support group participation
B. Encourage avoidance of social interaction
C. Focus only on medication adherence
D. Minimize emotional discussions

Q637. A patient with chronic GVHD complains of dry eyes and blurred vision. Which preventive measure is essential?

A. Frequent artificial tears
B. Rubbing eyes to stimulate tears
C. Using contact lenses daily
D. Skipping follow-up exams

Q638. A 37-year-old male survivor presents with elevated ferritin and transaminases. What is the likely cause?

A. Protein excess
B. Viral reactivation
C. Malnutrition
D. Transfusional iron overload

Q639. A patient reports thick, itchy rash and joint stiffness. Which therapy combination provides best results?

A. Topical steroids and physical therapy
B. Oral antibiotics and rest
C. Cooling lotion only
D. Extended bed rest

Q640. A 43-year-old HSCT survivor expresses fear of relapse despite remission. What should the nurse do first?

A. Provide emotional support and offer counseling referral
B. Minimize the concern to ease anxiety
C. Change topic to medical updates
D. Delay conversation until next visit

Q641. A 59-year-old survivor develops new skin lesions after prolonged sun exposure. What should the nurse emphasize?

A. Schedule dermatologic evaluation promptly

B. Increase sun exposure gradually
C. Delay exam until next check-up
D. Use tanning lotion to mask spots

Q642. A patient with hepatic GVHD asks about safe dietary habits. Which recommendation is best?
A. Skip vegetables and fruit
B. Increase high-fat meals for energy
C. Avoid alcohol and limit fatty foods
D. Use over-the-counter detox drinks

Q643. A survivor on tacrolimus develops mild tremors and rising creatinine. What does this indicate?
A. Tacrolimus toxicity
B. Iron overload
C. Steroid withdrawal
D. Viral nephritis

Q644. A patient reports persistent diarrhea three years post-HSCT. Stool studies are negative. What condition should be evaluated?
A. Chronic intestinal GVHD
B. Lactose intolerance
C. Irritable bowel syndrome
D. Acute viral infection

Q645. A survivor complains of fatigue and pallor. CBC shows low hemoglobin and high ferritin. What is the probable cause?
A. Iron overload anemia
B. Iron deficiency anemia
C. Vitamin deficiency anemia
D. Aplastic relapse

Q646. A 50-year-old patient reports blurry vision and difficulty reading fine print. Which complication is most likely?
A. Diabetic retinopathy
B. Bacterial conjunctivitis
C. Sinus infection
D. Radiation-induced cataract

Q647. A 44-year-old HSCT survivor presents with dry mouth and oral ulcers. What is the most likely cause?
A. Chronic oral GVHD
B. Vitamin B deficiency
C. Viral stomatitis
D. Gingivitis

Q648. A 57-year-old survivor experiences fatigue, low libido, and muscle weakness. Lab results show low testosterone. What is the likely cause?
A. Gonadal failure after conditioning therapy
B. Pituitary adenoma formation
C. Adrenal suppression from stress
D. Iron overload alone

Q649. A patient reports yellowing skin and elevated liver enzymes six months into chronic GVHD. Which organ system is involved?
A. Hepatic
B. Renal
C. Pulmonary

D. Gastrointestinal

Q650. A 40-year-old survivor reports fear of returning to work due to fatigue and immune risk. What should the nurse recommend?

A. Ignoring medical follow-up
B. Immediate full-time return
C. Permanent work avoidance
D. Gradual return with employer coordination and self-monitoring

Q651. A 38-year-old patient develops persistent cough and diffuse ground-glass opacities on CT 30 months after HSCT. What is the likely diagnosis?

A. Chronic pulmonary GVHD
B. Acute viral pneumonia
C. Pulmonary edema
D. Pleural effusion

Q652. A 60-year-old survivor reports recurrent infections and low immunoglobulin levels two years post-HSCT. What management is indicated?

A. Monthly IVIG infusions
B. Long-term antibiotic prophylaxis
C. Vitamin C supplementation
D. Increased protein diet

Q653. A 54-year-old survivor complains of skin dryness and restricted movement in hands. Which intervention helps most?

A. Regular stretching and emollient use
B. Heat packs alone
C. Prolonged rest
D. Increased corticosteroid dose

Q654. A survivor presents with persistent cough, fever, and multiple lung nodules. What late complication is most probable?

A. Bacterial tracheitis
B. Viral bronchitis
C. Fungal pneumonia
D. Pulmonary embolism

Q655. A patient reports easy bruising and fatigue three years post-HSCT. CBC shows thrombocytopenia. What should be evaluated?

A. Secondary marrow failure
B. Vitamin C deficiency
C. Drug allergy
D. Muscle wasting

Q656. A 46-year-old survivor reports chronic anxiety about cancer recurrence. What is the nurse's priority intervention?

A. Provide emotional support and refer to survivorship counseling
B. Advise ignoring anxiety
C. Recommend self-isolation
D. Defer discussion until later

Q657. Which factor most strongly influences long-term quality of life after hematopoietic stem cell transplantation (HSCT)?

A. Presence of chronic GVHD
B. Donor-recipient sex mismatch
C. Duration of hospital stay

D. Conditioning regimen type

Q658. A patient reports fatigue and difficulty concentrating six months post-transplant. What should the nurse assess first?

A. Level of exercise tolerance
B. Sleep habits only
C. Nutritional intake alone
D. Thyroid function and hemoglobin levels

Q659. Which intervention best supports coping and adjustment during early survivorship?

A. Participation in structured support groups
B. Avoidance of discussing illness
C. Self-isolation to prevent infection
D. Suppressing emotional expression

Q660. What is the most common long-term sexual health issue after HSCT?

A. Decreased libido and vaginal dryness
B. Priapism
C. Hypersexuality
D. Frequent infections

Q661. Which strategy best assists patients with chronic fatigue post-transplant?

A. Graded exercise and energy conservation
B. Extended daytime sleeping
C. Discontinuing activity completely
D. High-caffeine diet

Q662. What should be emphasized during education about returning to work after HSCT?

A. Avoid discussing limitations with employers
B. Immediate full-time return after discharge
C. Gradual reentry with flexible scheduling
D. Restrict all physical activity indefinitely

Q663. Which assessment tool is most appropriate for measuring post-transplant quality of life?

A. FACT-BMT (Functional Assessment of Cancer Therapy–Bone Marrow Transplant)
B. Beck Depression Inventory
C. Mini-Mental State Exam
D. SF-36 Physical Component only

Q664. What is a common psychosocial barrier for caregivers during the recovery phase?

A. Emotional exhaustion and role overload
B. Increased social engagement
C. Overreliance on professional staff
D. Diminished empathy

Q665. Which symptom is most associated with reduced social functioning after transplant?

A. Persistent fatigue
B. Improved appetite
C. Hair regrowth
D. Increased physical endurance

Q666. What primary concern should be discussed with pediatric HSCT survivors transitioning to adult care?

A. Employment stressors
B. Early retirement planning
C. Fertility preservation and late organ effects
D. Nutritional fads

Q667. Which intervention most effectively manages anxiety about relapse in long-term survivors?
A. Structured survivorship counseling
B. Avoidance of medical follow-up
C. Reassurance alone
D. Increased sedative use
Q668. A patient reports chronic dry eyes and mouth post-transplant. Which condition should be suspected?
A. Chronic GVHD with sicca symptoms
B. Acute GVHD
C. CMV reactivation
D. Vitamin deficiency
Q669. Which strategy promotes effective family adaptation during recovery?
A. Involving family in shared decision-making
B. Restricting discussion of prognosis
C. Limiting caregiver participation
D. Encouraging isolation for rest
Q670. What key topic should be covered in survivorship education before discharge?
A. Visitor policies
B. Hospital billing details
C. Long-term effects and lifestyle adjustments
D. Nutrition for weight loss
Q671. Which Chapter of functioning is most affected by prolonged corticosteroid therapy?
A. Physical endurance and muscle strength
B. Auditory perception
C. Fine motor coordination only
D. Visual acuity
Q672. What approach helps patients cope with uncertainty about relapse or late complications?
A. Mindfulness-based stress reduction programs
B. Avoiding medical discussions
C. Suppressing emotions
D. Using excessive reassurance
Q673. Which long-term effect can significantly limit independence in transplant survivors?
A. Chronic fatigue and muscle weakness
B. Improved mobility
C. Normalized blood counts
D. Resolved mucositis
Q674. What is the most appropriate nursing intervention to address body image concerns after HSCT?
A. Focus only on physical symptoms
B. Minimize discussion of appearance
C. Discourage use of wigs or cosmetics
D. Encourage participation in peer support and self-care activities
Q675. Which late complication requires multidisciplinary management for optimal quality of life?
A. Osteopenia secondary to corticosteroid therapy
B. Temporary nausea from medications
C. Mild appetite change
D. Reversible electrolyte imbalance
Q676. What is the nurse's primary goal when facilitating survivorship planning?
A. Promote autonomy and preparedness for self-management

B. Schedule frequent hospital visits indefinitely
C. Limit patient participation in decision-making
D. Focus only on medication schedules

Q677. Which symptom most impacts social reintegration after transplant?
A. Chronic fatigue
B. Mild cough
C. Hair loss
D. Dry skin

Q678. Which coping approach best reduces post-transplant anxiety?
A. Isolation rest
B. Strict silence
C. Guided imagery
D. Sedative use

Q679. Which intervention improves sleep quality in survivors?
A. Bedtime routine
B. Daytime naps
C. Late caffeine
D. Extended rest

Q680. Which factor most predicts delayed return to work?
A. Chronic GVHD
B. Donor age
C. Hair regrowth
D. Family support

Q681. What should be included in survivorship teaching?
A. Late effects
B. Daily meals
C. Visitor limits
D. Pain logs

Q682. Which exercise strategy is most effective post-transplant?
A. Short sprints
B. Intense lifting
C. Prolonged rest
D. Gradual walking

Q683. Which psychosocial service most benefits caregivers?
A. Support group
B. Extra rest
C. Reduced visits
D. Private time

Q684. Which symptom suggests steroid-induced muscle loss?
A. Weak legs
B. Facial rash
C. Sore throat
D. Hair thinning

Q685. Which intervention reduces fear of relapse?
A. Mindfulness
B. Distraction
C. Avoidance
D. Denial

Q686. Which factor most influences sexual satisfaction post-transplant?
A. Peer advice
B. Time delay
C. Open dialogue
D. Silence kept
Q687. Which approach enhances emotional resilience after HSCT?
A. Cognitive therapy
B. Daily news
C. Excess rest
D. Strict diet
Q688. Which assessment best measures fatigue impact?
A. Brief Fatigue
B. Daily pain
C. Fluid intake
D. Weight check
Q689. Which symptom requires referral to rehabilitation?
A. Persistent weakness
B. Minor nausea
C. Mild rash
D. Hair loss
Q690. Which education point helps prevent long-term complications?
A. Fast dieting
B. Strict rest
C. Routine exercise
D. Alcohol use
Q691. Which intervention addresses caregiver burnout?
A. Scheduled respite
B. Task increase
C. Emotional denial
D. Extended shifts
Q692. Which strategy fosters positive body image?
A. Peer support
B. Avoid mirrors
C. Ignore change
D. Hide scars
Q693. Which follow-up service improves late-life wellbeing?
A. Survivorship clinic
B. Emergency care
C. Temporary unit
D. Home nursing
Q694. Which health factor best predicts long-term vitality?
A. Appetite size
B. Hair regrowth
C. Skin tone
D. Physical activity
Q695. Which issue most commonly affects caregiver health?
A. Sleep loss
B. Weight gain

C. Hand tremor
D. Mild rash

Q696. Which long-term effect requires ongoing education?

A. Bone loss
B. Nail change
C. Hair dryness
D. Skin pallor

Q697. A 45-year-old patient, six months post-transplant, reports feeling isolated and avoids friends due to fatigue. What should the nurse recommend first?

A. Join support group
B. Limit visitors
C. Sleep longer
D. Avoid social events

Q698. A 28-year-old woman expresses anxiety about infertility after HSCT. What is the nurse's best action?

A. Suggest herbal remedy
B. Offer sedation
C. Delay discussion
D. Provide fertility referral

Q699. Which factor most predicts emotional distress in long-term survivors?

A. Chronic GVHD
B. Short hospital stay
C. Late meal timing
D. Improved stamina

Q700. A caregiver reports irritability and poor sleep. What should the nurse recommend?

A. Schedule respite
B. Increase duties
C. Limit counseling
D. Delay rest

Answer key and Explanation (601-700)
Q601. Answer: A
Explanation: Consistent moderate activity and balanced nutrition prevent vascular damage caused by radiation or steroids. Fat-rich diets, smoking, and erratic exercise elevate atherosclerotic and metabolic risk.
SubChapter: Cardiovascular Health – Prevention
Q602. Answer: C
Explanation: Mucosal GVHD causes immune-driven ulcerations resistant to antifungal therapy, requiring immunosuppression. Thrush shows white plaques, iron deficiency manifests as glossitis, and allergy reactions resolve rapidly after exposure cessation.
SubChapter: Oral Late Effects – GVHD
Q603. Answer: A
Explanation: Bone marrow suppression can recur late, presenting with thrombocytopenia and bleeding tendencies. Nutritional deficits cause anemia, allergic rash is pruritic, and dehydration does not produce bruising.
SubChapter: Hematologic Late Effects – Surveillance
Q604. Answer: A
Explanation: Infection prevention requires hygiene, mask use in crowds, and postponing live vaccines until immune recovery. Skipping boosters or follow-ups risks preventable illness and treatment gaps, and stopping prophylaxis may lead to relapse infections.
SubChapter: Immune Reconstitution – Education
Q605. Answer: A
Explanation: Tacrolimus may cause peripheral nerve irritation leading to paresthesia. Calcium deficiency results in cramps, fatigue is nonspecific, and myalgia affects muscles, not sensory nerves.
SubChapter: Pharmacologic Late Effects – Immunosuppressants
Q606. Answer: C
Explanation: Providing psychological counseling helps process fear, improve coping, and strengthen adjustment. Ignoring or postponing care deepens anxiety, while open discussion encourages proactive emotional management.
SubChapter: Psychosocial Support – Survivorship
Q607. Answer: A
Explanation: Chronic immune injury to small airways causes bronchiolitis obliterans, a hallmark late pulmonary complication in HSCT survivors. Asthma improves with bronchodilators, edema produces crackles not wheezing, and pneumonia causes acute fever and infiltrates.
SubChapter: Pulmonary Late Effects – Chronic GVHD
Q608. Answer: A
Explanation: Cardiovascular risk management through dietary modification and moderate exercise prevents metabolic syndrome post-HSCT. Fluid and protein restriction impair recovery, sodium elevation raises blood pressure, and inactivity increases cardiac risk.
SubChapter: Cardiovascular Health – Lifestyle
Q609. Answer: A
Explanation: Pulmonary fibrosis develops gradually due to chemotherapy or radiation-induced alveolar scarring. Acute infection and embolism cause sudden symptoms, and fluid overload presents with rapid weight gain and crackles.
SubChapter: Pulmonary Late Effects – Fibrotic
Q610. Answer: D

Explanation: Emotional adjustment requires counseling and structured re-engagement in normal roles. Avoidance or isolation worsens depression, and limiting support to medication neglects psychosocial rehabilitation.
SubChapter: Psychosocial & Emotional Recovery
Q611. Answer: A
Explanation: Radiation damages thyroid tissue, leading to hormone deficiency and slowed metabolism. Diabetes produces hyperglycemia, adrenal insufficiency causes hypotension, and hypoglycemia presents with tremors, not sustained weight gain.
SubChapter: Endocrine Late Effects – Thyroid
Q612. Answer: A
Explanation: Hepatic GVHD involves bile duct injury producing cholestatic enzyme elevation and itching. Viral hepatitis presents with transaminitis, renal failure alters creatinine, and gallstones cause transient obstruction rather than immune injury.
SubChapter: Hepatic Late Effects – GVHD
Q613. Answer: A
Explanation: Topical cyclosporine decreases ocular surface inflammation and restores lubrication in chronic GVHD. Redness drops mask symptoms, reduced hydration worsens dryness, and medication avoidance leads to corneal injury.
SubChapter: Ocular Late Effects – GVHD
Q614. Answer: C
Explanation: Morning dosing aligns with circadian rhythm, minimizing insomnia, while consistent sleep hygiene improves rest. Nighttime or missed doses destabilize control, and caffeine worsens irritability and insomnia.
SubChapter: Pharmacologic Late Effects – Corticosteroids
Q615. Answer: A
Explanation: Chelation removes excess iron accumulated from repeated transfusions, preventing hepatic and cardiac injury. Vitamin or diet changes do not reduce iron burden, and rest offers only temporary relief from systemic effects.
SubChapter: Metabolic Late Effects – Iron Overload
Q616. Answer: A
Explanation: Stretching prevents contractures and maintains range of motion in sclerotic GVHD. Immobility accelerates fibrosis, cold therapy gives short-term comfort only, and massage lacks sustained flexibility benefits.
SubChapter: Musculoskeletal Rehabilitation – GVHD
Q617. Answer: A
Explanation: Conditioning regimens damage ovarian follicles, resulting in irreversible menopause. Medication suppression resolves after therapy, stress alters cycles transiently, and infection scarring primarily affects tubes, not endocrine function.
SubChapter: Endocrine & Reproductive Late Effects
Q618. Answer: D
Explanation: Tacrolimus toxicity causes neuroexcitation and renal vasoconstriction, presenting as tremors and hypertension. Adrenal or anxiety conditions differ in etiology, and calcium imbalance does not provoke tremors.
SubChapter: Pharmacologic Late Effects – Immunosuppressants
Q619. Answer: A
Explanation: Structured counseling and peer survivorship groups improve coping and reduce post-traumatic stress. Isolation and avoidance reinforce distress, and focusing solely on physical recovery ignores psychological adaptation.

SubChapter: Psychosocial Late Effects – Adjustment

Q620. Answer: A

Explanation: Hypogammaglobulinemia impairs antibody defense, requiring immunoglobulin replacement for infection prevention. Chronic antibiotic or antihistamine use does not correct the deficiency, and nasal sprays treat local inflammation only.

SubChapter: Immune Reconstitution – Deficiency

Q621. Answer: A

Explanation: Rapid stiffness and skin changes suggest progressive GVHD requiring medical assessment and immunosuppressive adjustment. Topical or self-directed management delays treatment, and immobility increases contracture risk.

SubChapter: Musculoskeletal Late Effects – GVHD

Q622. Answer: D

Explanation: Saliva substitutes and gentle oral hygiene relieve xerostomia and maintain nutrition. Fluid restriction and high sodium aggravate dryness, while skipping dental visits heightens infection risk.

SubChapter: Oral Late Effects – Chronic GVHD

Q623. Answer: A

Explanation: Cognitive rehabilitation and structured training improve neuroplasticity and function after chemo- or radiation-related cognitive decline. Sedatives impair alertness, ignoring symptoms delays intervention, and isolation worsens deficits.

SubChapter: Neurocognitive Late Effects – Rehabilitation

Q624. Answer: A

Explanation: Immunosuppressed survivors are vulnerable to invasive fungal infections that manifest as nodules and low-grade fever. Viral bronchitis is self-limited, pneumonitis lacks nodules, and embolism presents abruptly with pleuritic pain.

SubChapter: Late Infectious Complications – Pulmonary

Q625. Answer: A

Explanation: Chronic steroid use increases lens opacity risk leading to cataract development. Retinal detachment and optic neuritis present acutely with pain, and glaucoma is gradual but more associated with intraocular pressure rise than direct lens clouding.

SubChapter: Ocular Late Effects – Pharmacologic

Q626. Answer: B

Explanation: Photosensitivity and skin cancer risk are elevated by immunosuppressants; sun protection and moderation are safest. Excess exposure aggravates lesions, halting therapy destabilizes GVHD, and complete avoidance reduces quality of life.

SubChapter: Dermatologic Late Effects – Education

Q627. Answer: A

Explanation: Bronchiolitis obliterans, a late noninfectious pulmonary GVHD manifestation, causes irreversible small airway obstruction. Pleural effusion produces fluid accumulation, embolism presents abruptly, and asthma typically improves with bronchodilators.

SubChapter: Pulmonary Late Effects – GVHD

Q628. Answer: A

Explanation: Gentle saline or bicarbonate rinses and saliva substitutes soothe mucosal inflammation and improve comfort. Alcohol-based rinses irritate tissues, acidic foods worsen pain, and skipping hygiene increases infection risk.

SubChapter: Oral Late Effects – Chronic GVHD

Q629. Answer: A

Explanation: Long-term corticosteroid therapy weakens bone density, causing fractures and pain. Calcium deficiency alone causes cramps, vitamin A excess affects liver function, and iron overload primarily impacts hepatic and cardiac systems.
SubChapter: Musculoskeletal Late Effects – Osteoporosis

Q630. Answer: D

Explanation: Gonadal toxicity from chemotherapy or irradiation reduces estrogen, causing infertility and menstrual changes. Cortisol and aldosterone regulate stress and electrolytes, and insulin governs glucose, not reproductive function.
SubChapter: Endocrine & Reproductive Late Effects

Q631. Answer: A

Explanation: Ursodeoxycholic acid improves bile flow and relieves cholestasis in hepatic GVHD. Antifungal and iron therapies are unrelated, while high-protein diets do not alleviate pruritus from biliary obstruction.
SubChapter: Hepatic Late Effects – GVHD

Q632. Answer: A

Explanation: Cognitive rehabilitation strengthens memory and attention in survivors with chemo- or radiation-induced cognitive impairment. Sedatives worsen focus, vitamins do not restore neurocognitive function, and social isolation reduces stimulation and adaptation.
SubChapter: Neurocognitive Late Effects – Rehabilitation

Q633. Answer: A

Explanation: Consistent low-intensity activity and emotional support improve energy and mood regulation. Prolonged rest exacerbates deconditioning, medication dependence ignores psychosocial components, and disregarding emotions delays holistic recovery.
SubChapter: Psychosocial & Physical Rehabilitation

Q634. Answer: D

Explanation: Moisturizers maintain elasticity, and stretching preserves joint motion in sclerotic GVHD. Restricting motion promotes contractures, alcohol gels irritate skin, and avoiding therapy reduces functional independence.
SubChapter: Musculoskeletal Late Effects – Sclerotic GVHD

Q635. Answer: A

Explanation: Steroid exposure and irradiation cause lens opacity, leading to cataract and light sensitivity. Optic neuritis involves pain and vision loss, detachment presents acutely, and conjunctivitis produces redness and discharge.
SubChapter: Ocular Late Effects – Pharmacologic

Q636. Answer: A

Explanation: Psychosocial rehabilitation and peer support mitigate post-transplant isolation and depression. Avoidance deepens emotional distress, limited care focus neglects mental health, and suppressing discussion impairs coping.
SubChapter: Psychosocial Late Effects – Social Reintegration

Q637. Answer: A

Explanation: Artificial tears preserve corneal integrity and reduce irritation in ocular GVHD. Rubbing increases damage, contact lens use worsens dryness, and avoiding follow-up misses progressive inflammation signs.
SubChapter: Ocular Late Effects – GVHD

Q638. Answer: D

Explanation: Frequent transfusions during treatment increase body iron stores, damaging hepatic tissue. Viral relapse raises transaminases but not ferritin, while nutrition imbalances do not account for both laboratory findings.

SubChapter: Metabolic Late Effects – Iron Overload
Q639. Answer: A
Explanation: Topical steroids reduce inflammation while physical therapy maintains mobility in sclerotic GVHD. Antibiotics treat infection, cooling lotions offer temporary comfort, and rest exacerbates contractures.
SubChapter: Dermatologic & Musculoskeletal Late Effects
Q640. Answer: A
Explanation: Addressing relapse fears through validation and counseling fosters coping and self-efficacy. Dismissing concerns or postponing discussion erodes trust and psychological resilience.
SubChapter: Psychosocial Late Effects – Fear of Recurrence
Q641. Answer: A
Explanation: Immunosuppressed patients face heightened risk of skin cancers; early assessment enables detection and treatment. Prolonged UV exposure and cosmetic concealment increase danger, and delays compromise outcomes.
SubChapter: Secondary Malignancies – Dermatologic
Q642. Answer: C
Explanation: Alcohol and fats aggravate liver inflammation; a balanced, low-fat diet supports hepatic recovery. High-fat intake or unverified detox regimens strain liver metabolism, while nutrient restriction reduces resilience.
SubChapter: Hepatic Late Effects – Education
Q643. Answer: A
Explanation: Tacrolimus can induce nephrotoxicity and neurotoxicity, shown by tremors and renal dysfunction. Iron overload and viral injury have distinct biochemical markers, while steroid withdrawal does not elevate creatinine.
SubChapter: Pharmacologic Late Effects – Immunosuppressants
Q644. Answer: A
Explanation: Chronic intestinal GVHD involves immune-mediated mucosal damage and poor absorption, leading to prolonged diarrhea. Lactose or IBS cause intermittent symptoms, and viral infections are acute.
SubChapter: Gastrointestinal Late Effects – GVHD
Q645. Answer: A
Explanation: Iron overload from transfusions can suppress erythropoiesis and cause fatigue despite high ferritin. Iron deficiency presents with low ferritin, vitamin deficiency causes macrocytosis, and relapse would reduce all cell lines.
SubChapter: Hematologic Late Effects – Metabolic
Q646. Answer: D
Explanation: Lens damage from total body irradiation or long-term steroids leads to cataract, impairing near vision. Conjunctivitis causes redness and discharge, sinus infection produces facial pressure, and diabetic retinopathy develops gradually with retinal vessel changes.
SubChapter: Ocular Late Effects – Radiation
Q647. Answer: A
Explanation: Chronic GVHD damages salivary glands, reducing secretion and causing ulcerations. Vitamin deficiency causes glossitis, viral stomatitis produces vesicular lesions, and gingivitis is limited to gum inflammation.
SubChapter: Oral Late Effects – GVHD
Q648. Answer: A

Explanation: Chemotherapy and irradiation damage gonadal tissue, reducing testosterone and leading to fatigue and weakness. Pituitary tumors are rare, stress-related adrenal suppression does not lower testosterone significantly, and iron overload primarily affects hepatic function.
SubChapter: Endocrine Late Effects – Gonadal

Q649. Answer: A

Explanation: Hepatic GVHD manifests with jaundice, elevated enzymes, and cholestasis. Renal involvement presents with creatinine elevation, pulmonary affects breathing, and gastrointestinal forms cause diarrhea rather than jaundice.
SubChapter: Hepatic Late Effects – GVHD

Q650. Answer: D

Explanation: A structured, gradual reintegration plan balances fatigue recovery and immune safety, improving confidence and adaptation. Abrupt return risks overexertion, avoidance promotes isolation, and skipping medical oversight endangers health stability.
SubChapter: Psychosocial Late Effects – Reintegration

Q651. Answer: A

Explanation: Chronic pulmonary GVHD presents with fibrotic and inflammatory airway injury producing diffuse opacities. Viral pneumonia is acute, pulmonary edema yields dependent infiltrates, and effusion causes fluid accumulation, not interstitial changes.
SubChapter: Pulmonary Late Effects – GVHD

Q652. Answer: A

Explanation: IV immunoglobulin replacement restores antibody levels and reduces infection risk in immune-deficient survivors. Antibiotics or diet changes do not correct antibody deficiency, and vitamins only enhance general wellness, not immune restoration.
SubChapter: Immune Reconstitution – Hypogammaglobulinemia

Q653. Answer: A

Explanation: Stretching and emollients preserve flexibility and reduce fibrosis in sclerotic GVHD. Heat therapy provides temporary relief, inactivity worsens contractures, and steroid escalation heightens systemic side effects without addressing mobility.
SubChapter: Musculoskeletal Late Effects – Sclerotic GVHD

Q654. Answer: C

Explanation: Immunosuppressed HSCT survivors are vulnerable to invasive fungal infections, often appearing as multiple nodules. Viral and bacterial infections are acute and less nodular, while embolism presents suddenly with chest pain and dyspnea.
SubChapter: Late Infectious Complications – Pulmonary

Q655. Answer: A

Explanation: Late marrow suppression results in thrombocytopenia and anemia, requiring prompt evaluation for relapse or secondary failure. Nutrient deficiency and drug allergy produce different symptoms, while muscle loss does not affect platelets.
SubChapter: Hematologic Late Effects – Surveillance

Q656. Answer: A

Explanation: Counseling and emotional validation help survivors address recurrence fears, promoting psychological resilience and adaptive coping. Ignoring or deferring discussion worsens anxiety, and isolation increases distress and social withdrawal.
SubChapter: Psychosocial Support – Survivorship Anxiety

Q657. Answer: A

Explanation: Chronic GVHD profoundly affects physical functioning, emotional wellbeing, and social participation, making it the leading determinant of long-term quality of life in HSCT survivors. Persistent symptoms can necessitate prolonged immunosuppression and limit rehabilitation efforts.

SubChapter: Long-Term Physical Health

Q658. Answer: D

Explanation: Fatigue and cognitive changes may result from anemia or thyroid dysfunction secondary to total body irradiation or medications. Screening laboratory values helps identify reversible causes before implementing behavioral interventions.

SubChapter: Physical and Cognitive Recovery

Q659. Answer: A

Explanation: Support groups facilitate normalization, shared experiences, and emotional expression, improving psychological adjustment post-transplant. Isolation and suppression delay recovery and increase anxiety and depression rates in survivors and caregivers.

SubChapter: Psychosocial Adaptation

Q660. Answer: A

Explanation: Hormonal alterations from chemotherapy and GVHD cause decreased libido, vaginal dryness, and erectile dysfunction. Addressing sexual health openly and providing hormonal or lubricating therapies enhance quality of life.

SubChapter: Sexual and Reproductive Health

Q661. Answer: A

Explanation: Gradual aerobic conditioning combined with rest planning reduces fatigue and enhances endurance. Over-sleeping and inactivity worsen deconditioning, while excessive caffeine disrupts restorative sleep patterns.

SubChapter: Physical Rehabilitation

Q662. Answer: C

Explanation: Phased return to work with flexible hours accommodates fluctuating stamina and medical follow-ups. Collaborative communication with employers promotes realistic goal setting and successful reintegration.

SubChapter: Vocational Reintegration

Q663. Answer: A

Explanation: The FACT-BMT specifically evaluates physical, emotional, and functional wellbeing in transplant recipients, capturing multidimensional recovery. Other tools measure isolated aspects like cognition or mood, lacking HSCT-specific sensitivity.

SubChapter: Quality-of-Life Measurement

Q664. Answer: A

Explanation: Family caregivers often experience burnout from continuous vigilance and emotional stress. Recognizing fatigue and offering respite or counseling supports sustained caregiving capacity and patient stability.

SubChapter: Caregiver Support

Q665. Answer: A

Explanation: Chronic fatigue limits participation in social, occupational, and recreational activities, impairing overall social reintegration. Symptom management and gradual physical conditioning improve engagement and perceived quality of life.

SubChapter: Physical and Social Functioning

Q666. Answer: C

Explanation: Pediatric survivors face long-term endocrine and fertility challenges requiring ongoing monitoring into adulthood. Early counseling ensures proactive management of reproductive and organ health risks.

SubChapter: Survivorship and Transition Care

Q667. Answer: A

Explanation: Counseling interventions provide coping strategies for uncertainty and reinforce adherence to monitoring schedules, improving emotional stability. Avoidance or sedation undermines psychological resilience and patient engagement.
SubChapter: Psychosocial Adaptation
Q668. Answer: A
Explanation: Chronic GVHD commonly affects exocrine glands, producing dryness in eyes and mouth similar to Sjögren-like syndrome. Early management prevents corneal injury and improves daily comfort.
SubChapter: Long-Term Physical Health
Q669. Answer: A
Explanation: Family engagement in decision-making fosters mutual understanding, decreases anxiety, and strengthens support systems, improving long-term adjustment. Withholding information increases mistrust and stress among caregivers.
SubChapter: Family-Centered Care
Q670. Answer: C
Explanation: Survivorship education ensures patients understand potential late effects, follow-up schedules, and necessary lifestyle modifications. Early preparation empowers patients and reduces anxiety about post-discharge independence.
SubChapter: Survivorship Education
Q671. Answer: A
Explanation: Long-term corticosteroid therapy leads to muscle wasting, weakness, and reduced physical stamina, diminishing daily function and quality of life. Early physiotherapy and nutritional support counteract deconditioning effects.
SubChapter: Physical Rehabilitation
Q672. Answer: A
Explanation: Mindfulness interventions help patients manage anxiety, improve sleep, and accept uncertainty. Avoidance or excessive reassurance delays psychological adaptation and self-efficacy in managing survivorship concerns.
SubChapter: Psychosocial Adaptation
Q673. Answer: A
Explanation: Persistent fatigue and muscle weakness hinder return to independent living and employment, requiring individualized rehabilitation plans to rebuild stamina and function. Monitoring progress maintains motivation and safety.
SubChapter: Physical and Social Functioning
Q674. Answer: D
Explanation: Supportive discussions and peer engagement help patients accept appearance changes such as alopecia or skin discoloration. Positive coping promotes self-esteem and psychosocial recovery.
SubChapter: Psychosocial Adaptation
Q675. Answer: A
Explanation: Corticosteroid-induced osteopenia necessitates collaboration between nursing, endocrinology, and rehabilitation teams to prevent fractures and maintain mobility. Multidisciplinary care ensures bone health and sustained activity.
SubChapter: Long-Term Physical Health
Q676. Answer: A
Explanation: Empowering survivors to self-manage health through education and autonomy enhances confidence, adherence, and life satisfaction. Over-dependence on the healthcare system hinders independence and transition to normalcy.
SubChapter: Survivorship Education
Q677. Answer: A

Explanation: Persistent fatigue reduces social participation, work engagement, and family involvement, making it a major obstacle to full reintegration after transplant. Energy-conservation techniques and progressive exercise restore endurance and confidence for social activities.
SubChapter: Physical and Social Functioning

Q678. Answer: C

Explanation: Guided imagery enhances relaxation and emotional regulation by redirecting attention away from distress. It supports adaptation and recovery, unlike isolation or excessive sedation, which may increase psychological distress and hinder resilience.
SubChapter: Psychosocial Adaptation

Q679. Answer: A

Explanation: Establishing consistent bedtime routines aligns circadian rhythm, reducing insomnia and fatigue common after transplant. Daytime naps or late caffeine disrupt restorative sleep cycles, worsening exhaustion and mood instability.
SubChapter: Physical Rehabilitation

Q680. Answer: A

Explanation: Chronic GVHD limits stamina and functional recovery through prolonged immunosuppression and physical discomfort. It remains the key predictor of delayed work resumption despite emotional and social readiness.
SubChapter: Vocational Reintegration

Q681. Answer: A

Explanation: Education about late complications such as endocrine, cardiovascular, and secondary cancer risks empowers patients to monitor and report symptoms early. Awareness promotes proactive, lifelong health management.
SubChapter: Survivorship Education

Q682. Answer: D

Explanation: Moderate walking programs rebuild endurance and reduce fatigue safely during immune recovery. Heavy lifting and inactivity increase injury or deconditioning risk, while sprinting strains recovering systems.
SubChapter: Physical Rehabilitation

Q683. Answer: A

Explanation: Support groups provide emotional validation, coping techniques, and shared experiences, reducing caregiver stress and isolation. While rest is helpful, structured support improves resilience and continuity of care.
SubChapter: Caregiver Support

Q684. Answer: A

Explanation: Prolonged corticosteroid use causes proximal muscle atrophy, especially in legs, leading to weakness and mobility decline. Early physiotherapy and nutritional support maintain strength and independence.
SubChapter: Long-Term Physical Health

Q685. Answer: A

Explanation: Mindfulness techniques help patients accept uncertainty, regulate emotion, and remain engaged with follow-up care. Avoidance and denial increase distress and reduce adherence to medical monitoring.
SubChapter: Psychosocial Adaptation

Q686. Answer: C

Explanation: Open discussion between partners and healthcare providers normalizes sexual concerns, allowing intervention for hormonal or emotional changes. Avoidance fosters shame and relationship strain.

SubChapter: Sexual and Reproductive Health
Q687. Answer: A
Explanation: Cognitive-behavioral therapy reframes negative thoughts, improving adjustment and hope during long-term recovery. Over-resting and rigid diets may worsen stress or body image concerns.
SubChapter: Psychosocial Adaptation
Q688. Answer: A
Explanation: The Brief Fatigue Inventory assesses intensity and interference with activities, guiding individualized management strategies. Routine pain or weight checks do not reflect functional fatigue burden accurately.
SubChapter: Physical and Social Functioning
Q689. Answer: A
Explanation: Lasting weakness suggests deconditioning that benefits from structured rehabilitation programs to restore strength and endurance. Minor transient symptoms resolve with standard supportive care.
SubChapter: Physical Rehabilitation
Q690. Answer: C
Explanation: Regular exercise maintains cardiovascular fitness and bone density, reducing risk of chronic complications after transplant. Prolonged rest and extreme diets impair recovery, while alcohol increases hepatic stress.
SubChapter: Long-Term Physical Health
Q691. Answer: A
Explanation: Planned respite provides essential rest and reduces emotional exhaustion for caregivers, preserving their long-term ability to support the patient. Overwork and denial accelerate burnout and compassion fatigue.
SubChapter: Caregiver Support
Q692. Answer: A
Explanation: Peer connections promote acceptance and self-confidence by sharing adaptive coping experiences. Avoidance behaviors heighten distress and social withdrawal, undermining psychological recovery.
SubChapter: Psychosocial Adaptation
Q693. Answer: A
Explanation: Dedicated survivorship clinics coordinate multidisciplinary care, monitor late effects, and promote ongoing quality-of-life improvement. Sporadic or acute services lack structured continuity needed for complex survivorship issues.
SubChapter: Survivorship and Transition Care
Q694. Answer: D
Explanation: Sustained physical activity improves stamina, reduces fatigue, and enhances psychological health in survivors. External appearance changes are less predictive of true functional vitality or wellbeing.
SubChapter: Physical Rehabilitation
Q695. Answer: A
Explanation: Sleep deprivation from constant caregiving leads to exhaustion, irritability, and reduced immune function. Prioritizing rest and external support sustains caregiver wellbeing and capacity.
SubChapter: Caregiver Support
Q696. Answer: A
Explanation: Corticosteroid and hormonal effects predispose survivors to osteopenia, requiring education on calcium intake, exercise, and monitoring. Early prevention maintains mobility and quality of life.

SubChapter: Long-Term Physical Health

Q697. Answer: A

Explanation: Joining a peer support group reduces isolation by fostering shared understanding and coping skills. Social connection encourages gradual reintegration and emotional recovery, improving overall quality of life.

SubChapter: Psychosocial Adaptation

Q698. Answer: D

Explanation: Prompt referral to fertility counseling enables informed decisions regarding preservation and hormonal therapy. Open discussion alleviates anxiety and enhances sense of control over reproductive health.

SubChapter: Sexual and Reproductive Health

Q699. Answer: A

Explanation: Chronic GVHD causes continuous symptom burden, visible changes, and dependency, increasing emotional distress. Comprehensive management and psychosocial support improve adaptation and resilience over time.

SubChapter: Long-Term Physical Health

Q700. Answer: A

Explanation: Scheduled respite provides rest and stress relief, preventing burnout and maintaining caregiving capacity. Overwork without support reduces performance and health, risking patient safety and family wellbeing.

SubChapter: Caregiver Support

Questions (701-800)

Q701. A patient complains of difficulty focusing at work after returning post-transplant. What initial step should be taken?

A. Assess cognitive changes
B. Recommend early retirement
C. Ignore complaint
D. Reduce hydration

Q702. Which brief intervention reduces nighttime anxiety and improves sleep?

A. Late exercise
B. Loud music
C. Bright lighting
D. Deep breathing

Q703. A 33-year-old man reports loss of sexual desire following transplant. What should the nurse address first?

A. Medication review
B. Peer advice
C. Fitness plan
D. Social media

Q704. Which statement reflects effective coping behavior?

A. "I walk daily and talk with friends."
B. "I stay in bed most days."
C. "I ignore my feelings."
D. "I avoid all visitors."

Q705. A 40-year-old HSCT recipient reports brittle bones after long steroid therapy. What preventive measure should the nurse reinforce?

A. Weight-bearing exercise
B. High-salt diet
C. Limited fluids
D. Sun avoidance

Q706. Which education topic supports long-term self-management?

A. Night shifts
B. Strict fasting
C. Rare follow-up
D. Regular screening

Q707. A patient feels guilty for depending on family assistance. What nursing response is best?

A. Normalize dependence
B. Suggest isolation
C. Encourage suppression
D. Ignore emotion

Q708. A nurse notices a patient refusing mirror views after hair loss. Which intervention is most therapeutic?

A. Encourage expression
B. Offer sedation
C. Avoid mirrors
D. Change topic

Q709. Which activity safely enhances endurance post-HSCT?

A. Light stretching

B. Heavy lifting
C. Long fasting
D. Intense sprints

Q710. A 50-year-old reports tingling and burning in hands months post-transplant. What should the nurse suspect?

A. Hypocalcemia
B. Skin GVHD
C. Peripheral neuropathy
D. Dehydration

Q711. Which scenario requires urgent psychosocial referral?

A. Survivor reports suicidal thoughts
B. Patient plans family trip
C. Caregiver requests day off
D. Patient joins exercise class

Q712. Which coping strategy helps children adapt after transplant?

A. Play therapy
B. Quiet isolation
C. Restrictive diet
D. Medication reward

Q713. A 47-year-old survivor reports severe fatigue limiting work. What collaborative referral is most helpful?

A. Physical therapy
B. Speech therapy
C. Dental clinic
D. Dermatology

Q714. What guidance improves adherence to follow-up care?

A. Late reminders
B. Verbal notes
C. Written plan
D. Phone calls only

Q715. A patient states, "I feel useless since the transplant." What is the most therapeutic response?

A. "Let's explore what gives meaning now."
B. "You must stay positive."
C. "Ignore that thought."
D. "It will pass soon."

Q716. Which intervention supports cognitive recovery after HSCT?

A. Memory training
B. Strict fasting
C. Long naps
D. Reduced reading

Q717. A 36-year-old survivor reports persistent sadness and poor appetite six months post-transplant. What is the nurse's best next step?

A. Screen for depression
B. Encourage more rest
C. Suggest herbal teas
D. Recommend exercise only

Q718. Which intervention supports patients who fear relapse during follow-up visits?

A. Reduced clinic visits

B. Extra medications
C. Mindfulness sessions
D. Avoided discussion

Q719. A 42-year-old caregiver reports guilt for losing patience with the patient. What should the nurse recommend?

A. Join support group
B. Increase workload
C. Limit counseling
D. Delay rest

Q720. Which factor most influences long-term emotional recovery after transplant?

A. Social support
B. Donor age
C. Hospital size
D. Meal timing

Q721. A 50-year-old patient complains of memory lapses after HSCT. What intervention is most effective?

A. Cognitive exercises
B. Extended naps
C. Reduced activity
D. Extra caffeine

Q722. Which education point promotes safe exercise after transplant?

A. Ignore fatigue cues
B. Train at high intensity
C. Avoid movement fully
D. Start light, progress slowly

Q723. A 29-year-old woman reports vaginal dryness after transplant. What should the nurse recommend?

A. Use lubricants
B. Increase fluids
C. Avoid intimacy
D. Take vitamins

Q724. Which finding requires immediate psychosocial referral?

A. Suicidal thoughts
B. Sleep delay
C. Mild fatigue
D. Appetite loss

Q725. A 40-year-old reports embarrassment over skin discoloration from GVHD. What should the nurse encourage?

A. Express feelings openly
B. Avoid mirrors completely
C. Limit social contact
D. Ignore emotional impact

Q726. Which factor is most associated with higher post-transplant fatigue?

A. Shorter stay
B. Younger age
C. Chronic GVHD
D. Donor type

Q727. What intervention helps manage steroid-induced weight gain?

A. Balanced diet plan
B. Strict fasting only
C. Avoid activity
D. Skip medications

Q728. A 35-year-old teacher struggles to resume work due to fatigue. What should the nurse recommend?

A. Gradual part-time return
B. Full-time return immediately
C. Avoid employment
D. Change profession

Q729. Which lifestyle choice best supports recovery after HSCT?

A. Regular exercise
B. Alcohol intake
C. Late meals
D. Tobacco use

Q730. A patient states, "I feel like my old self again." Which response shows effective adaptation?

A. "That's wonderful progress."
B. "Be careful not to overdo it."
C. "You might relapse again."
D. "Try not to feel that way."

Q731. Which health issue most limits quality of life in long-term survivors?

A. Small bruises
B. Minor rash
C. Hair loss
D. Chronic fatigue

Q732. What activity helps adolescents adjust after HSCT?

A. Peer mentorship
B. Limited school time
C. Strict home stay
D. Avoid communication

Q733. Which intervention addresses body image concerns effectively?

A. Counseling support
B. Ignore appearance
C. Avoid mirrors
D. Hide scars

Q734. Which routine health habit best prevents late complications?

A. Annual screenings
B. Irregular visits
C. Unrestricted diet
D. Skipped exercise

Q735. A 48-year-old survivor reports hand stiffness and skin thickening. What is the likely cause?

A. Fungal infection
B. Nutritional issue
C. Exercise strain
D. Chronic GVHD

Q736. Which caregiver behavior suggests burnout risk?

A. Irritability and insomnia
B. Joyful affect

C. Increased patience
D. Improved rest

Q737. A 52-year-old HSCT survivor reports difficulty concentrating at work. What nursing intervention is most appropriate?
A. Memory training
B. Longer breaks
C. More caffeine
D. Shorter shifts

Q738. Which patient report suggests positive adaptation to survivorship?
A. "I'm exercising again daily."
B. "I fear leaving home."
C. "I avoid social contact."
D. "I ignore my fatigue."

Q739. A 33-year-old caregiver says, "I can't handle this anymore." What immediate nursing response is most appropriate?
A. Provide reassurance
B. Offer new tasks
C. Delay counseling
D. Assess for burnout

Q740. Which factor most limits independence in long-term transplant survivors?
A. Chronic fatigue
B. Improved appetite
C. Clear skin
D. Normal vision

Q741. A 40-year-old survivor reports frustration over slow recovery. What should the nurse emphasize?
A. Progress takes time
B. Stop rehabilitation
C. Reduce follow-ups
D. Avoid goals

Q742. Which action most effectively supports healthy weight maintenance?
A. Balanced nutrition
B. Fad dieting
C. Skipping meals
D. High caffeine

Q743. A patient states, "I feel anxious before every checkup." What should the nurse recommend?
A. Delay visits
B. Skip appointments
C. Relaxation techniques
D. Request sedatives

Q744. Which finding suggests effective caregiver adaptation?
A. Accepts assistance
B. Refuses help
C. Avoids support
D. Suppresses emotion

Q745. A 46-year-old patient reports loss of interest in hobbies and social withdrawal. What should the nurse suspect?
A. Depression

B. Fatigue only
C. Medication side effect
D. Infection

Q746. Which approach promotes better adherence to medication regimens?
A. Verbal reminders
B. Written schedules
C. Sporadic timing
D. Visual avoidance

Q747. Which rehabilitation activity best aids gradual stamina recovery?
A. Walking program
B. Power lifting
C. Long fasting
D. Sleep extension

Q748. A 54-year-old reports difficulty enjoying meals due to altered taste. What is the best nursing recommendation?
A. Try flavor changes
B. Skip meals
C. Use sugar only
D. Avoid fluids

Q749. Which caregiver complaint signals need for professional help?
A. Sleep deprivation
B. Daily laughter
C. Improved patience
D. Good nutrition

Q750. A patient reports feeling disconnected from family months after recovery. What should the nurse suggest?
A. Limit visits
B. Family counseling
C. Ignore feelings
D. Avoid discussion

Q751. Which follow-up priority maintains long-term bone health?
A. Calcium intake
B. Caffeine use
C. Alcohol drinks
D. Low protein

Q752. Which education focus enhances independence after HSCT?
A. Self-care training
B. Task avoidance
C. Overprotection
D. Dependency

Q753. A 30-year-old man expresses fear of sexual intimacy after transplant. What should the nurse do first?
A. Assess concerns openly
B. Avoid discussion
C. Suggest medication
D. Delay topic

Q754. During a morbidity review, the team identifies delayed antibiotic initiation. The best QI approach is to:

A. Ignore
B. Blame
C. Root-cause
D. Delegate

Q755. Which practice most supports evidence-based nursing in transplant care?
A. Summarize research
B. Rely experience
C. Avoid change
D. Follow habit

Q756. For a unit seeking accreditation, the nurse manager's primary early task should be to:
A. Review standards
B. Hire staff
C. Fire staff
D. Paint walls

Q757. Which activity best reduces variability in chemotherapy administration processes?
A. Standardize
B. Improvise
C. Delay
D. Bypass

Q758. A nurse leader wants to track improvement after a handoff communication training. The most appropriate measure is:
A. Room size
B. Staff tenure
C. Handoff errors
D. Supply cost

Q759. When implementing a new survivorship pathway, best practice for stakeholder engagement is to:
A. Include clinicians
B. Exclude nurses
C. Forbid patients
D. Ignore staff

Q760. A run chart shows no improvement after interventions. Next step is to:
A. Reassess
B. Celebrate
C. Abandon
D. Punish

Q761. Which infection control practice is most impactful in reducing CLABSI in transplant units?
A. Max barrier
B. Faster discharge
C. No handwashing
D. More meds

Q762. A nurse documents a near-miss for wrong-rate infusion. This action primarily supports:
A. Secrecy
B. Litigation
C. Safety culture
D. Repetition

Q763. Which is the clearest indicator that a patient education program achieved learning outcomes?
A. Demonstration

B. Conversation
C. Pamphlet
D. Silence

Q764. A nurse manager wants to reduce medication error rates. Best first step is:
A. Audit med process
B. Blame nurses
C. Increase speed
D. Cut staffing

Q765. Which documentation practice most improves continuity of care during transfers?
A. Standardized note
B. Free-text only
C. Omit details
D. Delay entry

Q766. A unit introduces a checklist for discharge teaching. To ensure adoption, leader should:
A. Ignore feedback
B. Mandate silently
C. Remove checklist
D. Train staff

Q767. Which outcome best reflects success of a symptom-management pathway for GVHD?
A. Reduced ED visits
B. More emails
C. Longer stays
D. Increased billing

Q768. A nurse participates in a multidisciplinary morbidity conference. The most important behavior is to:
A. Share data
B. Stay silent
C. Defend only
D. Accuse others

Q769. Which method best evaluates patient satisfaction with survivorship services?
A. Validated survey
B. Verbal rumor
C. Anonymous insults
D. Ignore patients

Q770. Which action most strengthens staff resilience in a high-acuity transplant unit?
A. Reduce pay
B. Increase shifts
C. Limit breaks
D. Provide debriefs

Q771. During rounds, a nurse observes inconsistent hand hygiene among new staff. What should the charge nurse do first?
A. Educate staff
B. File complaint
C. Ignore behavior
D. Change roles

Q772. A 52-year-old patient's transfusion was delayed because consent was incomplete. Which quality improvement step addresses this issue long term?
A. Develop checklist

B. Increase staff
C. Reduce shifts
D. Skip consent

Q773. A nurse educator plans an in-service on evidence-based infection prevention. What should be emphasized first?
A. Guideline sources
B. Anecdotal cases
C. Staff stories
D. Unit gossip

Q774. A 38-year-old patient complains that discharge instructions were confusing. The nurse manager's first action should be to:
A. Repeat verbatim
B. Blame staff
C. Ignore issue
D. Audit teaching

Q775. Which practice best promotes ethical conduct in a BMT nursing team?
A. Maintain honesty
B. Delay truth
C. Hide data
D. Evade duty

Q776. A nurse leader notes staff burnout after several emergency admissions. What intervention supports professional well-being?
A. Peer debriefs
B. Ignore fatigue
C. Add workload
D. Limit breaks

Q777. A nurse identifies a pattern of late lab reporting affecting treatment schedules. Which QI tool is best?
A. Process map
B. Staff memo
C. Complaint form
D. Informal talk

Q778. A patient developed a preventable central line infection. During RCA, what must the team avoid?
A. Reviewing steps
B. Finding cause
C. Assigning blame
D. Collecting data

Q779. A unit tracks readmission rates monthly. What does this measure reflect?
A. Care continuity
B. Room turnover
C. Staff age
D. Visitor hours

Q780. A new nurse witnesses a medication error but hesitates to report it. The mentor should emphasize:
A. Nonpunitive culture
B. Harsher penalties
C. Peer silence

D. Delay reporting

Q781. During a policy revision, what ensures updated protocols remain practical?

A. Staff input
B. External ads
C. Management-only edits
D. Random polls

Q782. A nurse notes inconsistent premedication for transplant infusions. Which first action supports quality improvement?

A. Delay review
B. Skip dose
C. Avoid reporting
D. Verify order

Q783. A nurse-led project aims to reduce transfusion errors. Which measure best evaluates success?

A. Error rate
B. Bed count
C. Budget use
D. Staff age

Q784. A nurse educator plans to teach handoff communication using SBAR. What outcome confirms success?

A. Fewer miscommunications
B. More paperwork
C. Extra shifts
D. Silence at report

Q785. During patient care rounds, the physician dismisses a nurse's observation of early sepsis signs. The nurse's next best step is to:

A. Advocate again
B. Stay silent
C. Leave room
D. File grievance

Q786. The transplant unit initiates a new protocol for double-checking chemotherapy doses. What is this process primarily designed to reduce?

A. Supply shortage
B. Staff turnover
C. Medication error
D. Patient wait time

Q787. A patient's caregiver reports that discharge instructions vary among nurses. What action should leadership take?

A. Standardize education
B. Ignore complaints
C. Replace staff
D. Limit teaching

Q788. A nurse manager receives multiple reports of delayed blood draws. The best initial intervention is to:

A. Observe workflow
B. Punish staff
C. Ignore delays
D. Cancel draws

Q789. A nurse proposes implementing an electronic incident reporting tool. Which benefit should be emphasized to gain staff buy-in?
A. Easier reporting
B. Longer forms
C. Limited access
D. More paperwork
Q790. A nurse observes inconsistent donning of PPE during isolation care. Which strategy sustains long-term improvement?
A. Ignore errors
B. One-time memo
C. Ongoing audits
D. Reduce training
Q791. A nurse observes that timeouts before central line insertions are skipped during busy hours. What should the charge nurse do first?
A. Reinforce protocol
B. Ignore situation
C. Shorten timeouts
D. Report anonymously
Q792. A 60-year-old post-HSCT patient is readmitted within five days due to medication confusion. What system improvement best prevents recurrence?
A. Simplify instructions
B. Extend visits
C. Add medications
D. Remove labels
Q793. A nurse manager is planning a unit audit to assess documentation accuracy. What is the primary goal?
A. Identify trends
B. Punish errors
C. Hide findings
D. Reduce entries
Q794. A 45-year-old nurse struggles to manage heavy workload during increased census. The most appropriate leadership response is to:
A. Ignore stress
B. Criticize staff
C. Delay breaks
D. Adjust assignments
Q795. A new nurse fails to follow a sterile dressing protocol. The educator's most effective corrective action is to:
A. Demonstrate correctly
B. Assign punishment
C. Ignore incident
D. Delay feedback
Q796. Which nursing action best demonstrates professional accountability?
A. Admit error
B. Hide mistake
C. Shift blame
D. Delay report

Q797. A 55-year-old patient reports receiving conflicting dietary advice from different staff. What improvement approach should the nurse manager apply?

A. Standardize education

B. Rotate instructors

C. Delay response

D. Cancel sessions

Q798. A nurse leading a unit-based project on hand hygiene compliance should start with which activity?

A. Ignore data

B. Train randomly

C. Punish errors

D. Collect baseline

Q799. During multidisciplinary rounds, a disagreement arises about patient isolation needs. The nurse's best role is to:

A. Present evidence

B. Stay silent

C. Pick sides

D. Leave room

Q800. A nurse leader evaluates compliance with chemotherapy verification. What outcome indicates successful improvement?

A. Zero mismatches

B. Faster charting

C. Fewer breaks

D. Higher volume

Answer key and Explanation (701-800)

Q701. Answer: A

Explanation: Neurocognitive assessment helps identify attention or memory deficits from therapy or medications. Targeted cognitive rehabilitation and workplace accommodations promote successful reintegration.

SubChapter: Cognitive Recovery

Q702. Answer: D

Explanation: Deep-breathing relaxation techniques lower stress hormones, easing sleep initiation and quality. Environmental stimulation like noise or exercise close to bedtime disrupts circadian rhythm and increases fatigue.

SubChapter: Physical Rehabilitation

Q703. Answer: A

Explanation: Certain medications and hormonal changes impair libido; reviewing drugs and hormonal function guides appropriate interventions. Emotional counseling and partner communication follow pharmacologic assessment.

SubChapter: Sexual and Reproductive Health

Q704. Answer: A

Explanation: Active lifestyle and social engagement signify adaptive coping, enhancing mood and self-efficacy. Avoidance and isolation worsen depression and limit quality-of-life improvement.

SubChapter: Psychosocial Adaptation

Q705. Answer: A

Explanation: Weight-bearing activity stimulates bone formation and prevents steroid-induced osteoporosis. Dietary balance with calcium and vitamin D further preserves bone health and independence.

SubChapter: Long-Term Physical Health

Q706. Answer: D

Explanation: Routine follow-up and screenings detect late organ toxicity, metabolic disorders, and secondary cancers early. Consistent health surveillance enhances longevity and quality of life post-transplant.

SubChapter: Survivorship Education

Q707. Answer: A

Explanation: Validating dependence as part of recovery alleviates guilt and promotes emotional healing. Normalization reduces shame, allowing the patient to accept help and rebuild autonomy gradually.

SubChapter: Psychosocial Adaptation

Q708. Answer: A

Explanation: Allowing patients to express appearance concerns fosters acceptance and adaptation. Supportive dialogue and coping strategies restore body image confidence. Avoidance prolongs emotional distress.

SubChapter: Psychosocial Adaptation

Q709. Answer: A

Explanation: Low-impact stretching promotes gradual strength restoration without overexertion. Progressive conditioning prevents fatigue and deconditioning common in post-transplant recovery.

SubChapter: Physical Rehabilitation

Q710. Answer: C

Explanation: Chemotherapy and immunosuppressants can cause peripheral neuropathy, affecting sensory and motor function. Early recognition and pharmacologic management reduce discomfort and functional limitation.

SubChapter: Long-Term Physical Health

Q711. Answer: A
Explanation: Suicidal ideation signals severe psychological distress requiring immediate mental-health intervention. Rapid referral ensures safety and provides crisis stabilization and long-term therapy resources.
SubChapter: Psychosocial Adaptation
Q712. Answer: A
Explanation: Play therapy allows emotional expression and understanding in pediatric patients, easing fear and anxiety about treatment and body changes. Isolation intensifies distress and delays recovery.
SubChapter: Psychosocial Adaptation
Q713. Answer: A
Explanation: Physical therapy provides graded exercise and endurance training, improving strength and decreasing fatigue. It restores functional independence essential for occupational reintegration.
SubChapter: Physical Rehabilitation
Q714. Answer: C
Explanation: Written individualized care plans enhance understanding and retention, promoting adherence to monitoring schedules. Documentation provides clarity and accountability for both patient and team.
SubChapter: Survivorship Education
Q715. Answer: A
Explanation: Exploring meaning encourages self-reflection and purpose reconstruction, fostering emotional healing and post-traumatic growth. Dismissing feelings invalidates experience and increases hopelessness.
SubChapter: Psychosocial Adaptation
Q716. Answer: A
Explanation: Cognitive rehabilitation, including memory and attention exercises, mitigates chemo-brain symptoms and enhances daily functioning. Structured stimulation restores confidence in mental performance.
SubChapter: Cognitive Recovery
Q717. Answer: A
Explanation: Persistent sadness and appetite loss are hallmark symptoms of depression. Screening identifies psychological distress early, allowing timely referral for therapy or medication. Addressing mental health improves overall recovery and functioning.
SubChapter: Psychosocial Adaptation
Q718. Answer: C
Explanation: Mindfulness training fosters calm awareness of fears, helping patients manage uncertainty without avoidance. It decreases anxiety and encourages continued engagement in care and survivorship planning.
SubChapter: Psychosocial Adaptation
Q719. Answer: A
Explanation: Caregiver guilt and burnout respond well to structured support groups that normalize emotions and teach coping strategies. Peer validation and guided discussion rebuild confidence and emotional balance.
SubChapter: Caregiver Support
Q720. Answer: A
Explanation: Consistent social and emotional support is the strongest predictor of long-term psychological wellbeing post-transplant. Family involvement, peer connection, and counseling reduce depression and foster adaptation.
SubChapter: Psychosocial Adaptation

Q721. Answer: A
Explanation: Structured cognitive exercises enhance concentration, attention, and recall. They help counter chemotherapy-related cognitive impairment ("chemo brain") and improve daily performance. Rest alone rarely reverses memory issues.
SubChapter: Cognitive Recovery
Q722. Answer: D
Explanation: Gradual, progressive exercise minimizes fatigue and supports cardiac and muscular recovery without overexertion. Ignoring body cues increases injury and delays rehabilitation.
SubChapter: Physical Rehabilitation
Q723. Answer: A
Explanation: Vaginal dryness is a common consequence of estrogen deficiency post-HSCT. Water-based lubricants or topical estrogen therapy restore comfort and maintain relationship intimacy.
SubChapter: Sexual and Reproductive Health
Q724. Answer: A
Explanation: Suicidal ideation signals severe depression and mandates urgent referral for psychiatric evaluation and crisis support. Prompt action ensures patient safety and stabilizes mental health outcomes.
SubChapter: Psychosocial Adaptation
Q725. Answer: A
Explanation: Encouraging expression of appearance-related distress validates emotions and supports adjustment. Discussion allows introduction of supportive counseling and cosmetic resources that enhance confidence.
SubChapter: Psychosocial Adaptation
Q726. Answer: C
Explanation: Chronic GVHD prolongs systemic inflammation and immunosuppressive therapy, significantly increasing fatigue and limiting daily functioning. Managing GVHD symptoms and structured rehabilitation restore stamina.
SubChapter: Long-Term Physical Health
Q727. Answer: A
Explanation: Balanced diet with portion control and consistent mild exercise mitigates corticosteroid-related weight gain and metabolic complications. Abrupt medication changes endanger stability and graft survival.
SubChapter: Long-Term Physical Health
Q728. Answer: A
Explanation: Phased reentry with part-time scheduling allows adaptation to physical and cognitive demands, supporting endurance and success in work reintegration. Abrupt return increases exhaustion risk.
SubChapter: Vocational Reintegration
Q729. Answer: A
Explanation: Regular physical activity enhances mood, immunity, and cardiovascular health post-transplant, promoting holistic recovery. Substance use and poor nutrition delay healing and increase late-effect risks.
SubChapter: Physical Rehabilitation
Q730. Answer: A
Explanation: Positive reinforcement of emotional and physical recovery encourages continued self-care and resilience. Recognizing achievement validates progress and supports confidence in survivorship.
SubChapter: Psychosocial Adaptation
Q731. Answer: D

Explanation: Persistent fatigue affects mobility, independence, and mood more than cosmetic or minor symptoms, making it the predominant barrier to full quality-of-life restoration.
SubChapter: Physical and Social Functioning

Q732. Answer: A

Explanation: Peer mentorship connects adolescents with others who understand transplant experiences, reducing isolation and promoting healthy psychosocial adjustment. Restrictive isolation increases withdrawal and anxiety.
SubChapter: Psychosocial Adaptation

Q733. Answer: A

Explanation: Counseling provides coping strategies and confidence-building approaches to manage body image changes post-HSCT. It supports reintegration and emotional healing.
SubChapter: Psychosocial Adaptation

Q734. Answer: A

Explanation: Annual multidisciplinary evaluations detect late organ toxicities and secondary malignancies early. Regular screening and lifestyle maintenance sustain long-term health.
SubChapter: Survivorship Education

Q735. Answer: D

Explanation: Chronic GVHD can cause scleroderma-like skin changes, restricting mobility and daily activities. Early therapy with topical agents and physiotherapy reduces progression and discomfort.
SubChapter: Long-Term Physical Health

Q736. Answer: A

Explanation: Irritability, sleep loss, and emotional exhaustion indicate caregiver fatigue. Recognizing these signs allows timely intervention through counseling, respite care, and stress management.
SubChapter: Caregiver Support

Q737. Answer: A

Explanation: Memory training and cognitive exercises effectively address attention and focus deficits known as “chemo brain.” They enhance task performance, confidence, and daily productivity, improving overall quality of life after HSCT.
SubChapter: Cognitive Recovery

Q738. Answer: A

Explanation: Resuming structured activity demonstrates psychological readiness, restored stamina, and positive adaptation. Physical exercise improves energy, mood, and confidence in survivors, reinforcing recovery momentum.
SubChapter: Psychosocial Adaptation

Q739. Answer: D

Explanation: Emotional exhaustion and hopelessness indicate caregiver burnout. Prompt assessment identifies severity and triggers early interventions such as respite care or psychological support to prevent health decline and maintain caregiving quality.
SubChapter: Caregiver Support

Q740. Answer: A

Explanation: Persistent fatigue limits daily functioning, employment, and participation in social activities. Targeted rehabilitation and energy conservation strategies are crucial to restoring independence and enhancing self-efficacy post-transplant.
SubChapter: Physical and Social Functioning

Q741. Answer: A

Explanation: Normalizing gradual recovery expectations reduces frustration and promotes sustained engagement in rehabilitation. Encouragement builds motivation, fostering realistic optimism and long-term adherence to recovery plans.

SubChapter: Psychosocial Adaptation

Q742. Answer: A

Explanation: Balanced diets with adequate protein and micronutrients sustain muscle mass and energy while preventing metabolic complications. Extreme diets or stimulant use destabilize recovery and nutrient balance.

SubChapter: Long-Term Physical Health

Q743. Answer: C

Explanation: Relaxation methods such as deep breathing and mindfulness reduce anticipatory anxiety and encourage continued participation in follow-up care. Avoidance reinforces fear and undermines survivorship engagement.

SubChapter: Psychosocial Adaptation

Q744. Answer: A

Explanation: Accepting help demonstrates healthy coping and understanding of personal limits. It sustains caregiving endurance and improves family dynamics during the prolonged transplant recovery phase.

SubChapter: Caregiver Support

Q745. Answer: A

Explanation: Anhedonia and social isolation are characteristic signs of depression in HSCT survivors. Early screening and mental-health referral prevent worsening and promote psychosocial restoration.

SubChapter: Psychosocial Adaptation

Q746. Answer: B

Explanation: Written medication plans enhance consistency and reduce forgetfulness, especially for survivors managing complex regimens. Structured documentation fosters accountability and patient confidence.

SubChapter: Survivorship Education

Q747. Answer: A

Explanation: Progressive walking safely rebuilds cardiovascular endurance and muscle tone, combating deconditioning without strain. It is widely recommended in early post-transplant rehabilitation plans.

SubChapter: Physical Rehabilitation

Q748. Answer: A

Explanation: Experimenting with varied seasonings and temperatures helps overcome dysgeusia from conditioning therapy. Adaptation encourages adequate nutrition and enjoyment in eating.

SubChapter: Long-Term Physical Health

Q749. Answer: A

Explanation: Chronic sleep loss indicates significant stress and fatigue in caregivers, impairing judgment and health. Professional intervention and respite programs restore balance and prevent burnout.

SubChapter: Caregiver Support

Q750. Answer: B

Explanation: Family counseling restores communication and redefines roles disrupted by illness. Guided therapy rebuilds connection and shared understanding, improving relational quality post-transplant.

SubChapter: Family-Centered Care

Q751. Answer: A

Explanation: Adequate calcium intake, along with vitamin D and weight-bearing exercise, prevents osteopenia and maintains skeletal strength after corticosteroid therapy.

SubChapter: Long-Term Physical Health

Q752. Answer: A

Explanation: Teaching self-management fosters confidence, responsibility, and autonomy in survivors transitioning to independent living. Overprotection hinders growth and self-efficacy development.

SubChapter: Survivorship Education

Q753. Answer: A

Explanation: Open assessment normalizes sensitive discussions and identifies physical or emotional barriers to intimacy. Communication builds trust and guides appropriate interventions.

SubChapter: Sexual and Reproductive Health

Q754. Answer: C

Explanation: Root-cause analysis systematically uncovers system, process, and human factors leading to delay, enabling corrective system-level changes. Blame discourages reporting, ignoring perpetuates harm, and delegation without analysis risks superficial fixes. Root-cause fosters sustainable improvement and staff engagement.

SubChapter: Event Analysis & Improvement

Q755. Answer: A

Explanation: Summarizing applicable research and translating findings into local protocols supports evidence-based practice. Reliance on experience alone, resisting change, or habit-driven care can perpetuate outdated practices. Evidence synthesis combined with local adaptation improves outcomes and standardizes high-quality care.

SubChapter: Evidence-Based Practice

Q756. Answer: A

Explanation: Early review of accreditation standards identifies documentation, policy, staffing, and outcome requirements and frames a gap analysis. Hiring or staffing changes follow identified needs; cosmetic changes are irrelevant. Standards review enables prioritized action plans and timeline creation for compliance.

SubChapter: Accreditation & Regulatory Prep

Q757. Answer: A

Explanation: Standardizing protocols (checklists, double-checks, preprinted orders) reduces variation and medication errors. Improvisation and bypassing procedures increase risk, and delays compromise timely care. Standardization with staff input increases adherence and improves safety in complex transplant regimens.

SubChapter: Process Standardization & Safety

Q758. Answer: C

Explanation: Tracking handoff-related errors or communication incidents directly measures training impact. Staff tenure, room size, and supply cost are unrelated to communication effectiveness. Use pre/post metrics, audits, and staff surveys to evaluate sustained change and identify reinforcement needs.

SubChapter: Communication & Handoffs

Q759. Answer: A

Explanation: Inclusive engagement of clinicians, nurses, allied health, and patients ensures pathways are feasible, patient-centered, and implementable. Excluding key stakeholders or patients undermines acceptability and sustainability. Co-design fosters ownership and smoother adoption across multidisciplinary teams.

SubChapter: Change Management & Teamwork

Q760. Answer: A

Explanation: Lack of improvement prompts reassessment of intervention fidelity, measurement accuracy, root causes, and contextual barriers. Celebration is premature, abandonment wastes resources, and punitive responses harm team morale. Reassessment refines the approach with Plan-Do-Study-Act cycles.

SubChapter: Data-Driven QI Cycles

Q761. Answer: A

Explanation: Maximal sterile barrier precautions during central line insertion and strict maintenance protocols reduce CLABSI. Faster discharge and more medications are not primary prevention strategies, and forgoing hand hygiene increases infection risk. Maintenance bundles plus staff training sustain reductions.
SubChapter: Infection Prevention & Bundles
Q762. Answer: C
Explanation: Reporting near-misses fosters a culture of safety, enabling system fixes before harm occurs. Concealment impedes learning, and litigation focus is secondary. Transparent reporting coupled with analysis demonstrates organizational commitment to continuous improvement.
SubChapter: Safety Culture & Reporting
Q763. Answer: A
Explanation: Patient demonstration of skill (e.g., port care, medication administration) objectively shows competency and learning. Conversation alone may be superficial, pamphlets passive, and silence ambiguous. Demonstration with return-teach methods and documentation ensures readiness for self-care.
SubChapter: Patient Education & Competency
Q764. Answer: A
Explanation: Auditing the medication process identifies error points (ordering, dispensing, administration), enabling targeted interventions like barcode scanning, education, and process redesign. Blame, speed-up, or staffing cuts worsen safety. Data-driven audits guide effective corrective actions.
SubChapter: Medication Safety
Q765. Answer: A
Explanation: Standardized transfer notes ensure critical information (allergies, meds, lines, recent events) is reliably communicated. Free-text without structure risks omissions; omitting details or delaying entries threatens patient safety during transitions. Structured templates enhance clarity and auditability.
SubChapter: Documentation & Transitions
Q766. Answer: D
Explanation: Training, role modeling, and allowing staff input on checklist content promote adoption and meaningful use. Silent mandates or ignoring feedback reduce buy-in; removing tools stops improvement. Ongoing audit and refinement maintain relevance and compliance.
SubChapter: Implementation & Sustainment
Q767. Answer: A
Explanation: Reduced emergency visits and urgent admissions indicate effective outpatient symptom control and timely intervention. Increased communications or billing may reflect activity but not improved patient outcomes; longer stays usually signal deterioration rather than pathway success.
SubChapter: Outcome Selection & Measurement
Q768. Answer: A
Explanation: Sharing accurate data and observations promotes objective learning and system improvement. Defensive or accusatory behavior undermines collaborative problem-solving. Constructive participation focuses on system fixes, not personal blame, fostering a learning culture that reduces future harm.
SubChapter: Team Reviews & Professionalism
Q769. Answer: A
Explanation: Validated patient-reported outcome measures capture satisfaction and unmet needs reliably, allowing benchmarking and targeted improvements. Informal rumors lack rigor, insults are unstructured, and ignoring feedback forfeits opportunities to enhance patient-centered care.
SubChapter: Patient Experience Measurement

Q770. Answer: D
Explanation: Regular debriefings, access to mental health resources, workload balancing, and recognition build resilience and reduce burnout. Increasing shifts or limiting breaks exacerbates stress, and punitive financial changes demoralize staff. Proactive support sustains workforce performance and retention.
SubChapter: Workforce Wellbeing & Retention
Q771. Answer: A
Explanation: Immediate bedside education reinforces standards and corrects unsafe practices without delay. Filing complaints prematurely discourages openness, ignoring issues normalizes risk, and role changes address symptoms, not causes. Education ensures safety compliance through real-time reinforcement.
SubChapter: Infection Control & Practice Coaching
Q772. Answer: A
Explanation: Introducing a standardized pre-transfusion checklist ensures consent completion, specimen verification, and timely workflow. Staffing or schedule changes may not fix process gaps, and skipping consent violates ethical and regulatory standards. Structured checklists prevent omission errors effectively.
SubChapter: Process Improvement – Safety
Q773. Answer: A
Explanation: Starting with credible evidence sources (CDC, EBMT, institutional guidelines) validates content and promotes best-practice adoption. Anecdotes and gossip distract from standardized knowledge and weaken credibility. Reference-based education builds professional competence and accountability.
SubChapter: Evidence-Based Education
Q774. Answer: D
Explanation: Auditing education documentation and observing teaching reveals process deficiencies and comprehension barriers. Blame erodes trust, ignoring misses improvement opportunity, and repetition without revision fails to address the root cause. Auditing enables targeted redesign of materials.
SubChapter: Patient Education Quality
Q775. Answer: A
Explanation: Honesty builds patient trust, team cohesion, and ethical decision-making in transplant settings. Withholding truth or manipulating data undermines professionalism and may compromise care integrity. Transparency ensures accountability and upholds ethical standards.
SubChapter: Ethical Nursing Practice
Q776. Answer: A
Explanation: Peer debriefings normalize stress discussion, enhance coping, and reduce long-term burnout risk. Ignoring symptoms or increasing workload worsens fatigue; limiting breaks impairs focus. Structured recovery sessions sustain team resilience and safety.
SubChapter: Workforce Support & Resilience
Q777. Answer: A
Explanation: Process mapping visualizes workflow delays and identifies systemic bottlenecks. Memos or complaints communicate issues but don't clarify causes; informal discussion lacks actionable structure. Process mapping guides redesigns and measurable change in turnaround times.
SubChapter: Quality Improvement Tools
Q778. Answer: C
Explanation: Root cause analysis should focus on systemic factors and preventive redesigns, not individual blame. Blame suppresses reporting and learning. Collecting data and reviewing process steps are constructive RCA components fostering safety culture.

SubChapter: Root Cause Analysis

Q779. Answer: A

Explanation: Readmission rate indicates effectiveness of discharge planning, patient education, and continuity of care. Room turnover and staff demographics do not measure quality outcomes; visitor schedules are irrelevant. Tracking readmissions identifies areas needing stronger follow-up.

SubChapter: Quality Outcome Monitoring

Q780. Answer: A

Explanation: A nonpunitive environment encourages transparent reporting for learning and system correction. Punitive or silent responses perpetuate underreporting. Immediate, supportive feedback reinforces accountability and safety awareness within a trust-based culture.

SubChapter: Safety Culture & Reporting

Q781. Answer: A

Explanation: Involving bedside nurses ensures new protocols are feasible, relevant, and aligned with actual workflows. Exclusive management control risks impractical designs; random surveys without context lack depth. Collaborative updates enhance compliance and sustainability.

SubChapter: Policy Development & Engagement

Q782. Answer: D

Explanation: Verifying premedication orders ensures safety and clarifies workflow inconsistencies before error reporting or corrective redesign. Avoiding documentation or delay endangers patients; dose omission violates safe practice. Verification ensures alignment with standard protocols.

SubChapter: Safe Medication Practice

Q783. Answer: A

Explanation: Reduction in transfusion error rate directly measures project effectiveness. Bed count and staff demographics do not reflect safety improvement, while budget monitoring tracks resources, not outcome. Outcome-based evaluation validates intervention impact.

SubChapter: Performance Metrics

Q784. Answer: A

Explanation: Reduced miscommunication events validate SBAR training success, showing improved structure and clarity in transitions. Paperwork and shift volume are unrelated, and silence may reflect disengagement, not improvement. Regular audits confirm sustained practice adoption.

SubChapter: Communication & Handoff Safety

Q785. Answer: A

Explanation: Persistent, respectful advocacy ensures patient safety and fulfills the nurse's duty to prevent harm. Silence or avoidance risks delay in treatment. Grievance may follow if concerns are ignored but should not replace immediate advocacy.

SubChapter: Professional Advocacy

Q786. Answer: C

Explanation: Independent double-checking is a proven strategy to intercept chemotherapy dosing errors. Staff retention and logistics are unaffected directly, and wait time changes are incidental. Safety redundancy significantly lowers high-risk medication incidents.

SubChapter: Medication Safety & Verification

Q787. Answer: A

Explanation: Developing standardized teaching checklists ensures consistent content, reduces confusion, and supports patient safety. Ignoring concerns or restricting teaching weakens quality, while replacement addresses individuals rather than systemic inconsistency.

SubChapter: Patient Education Standardization

Q788. Answer: A

Explanation: Direct workflow observation reveals systemic barriers—supply issues, timing, or communication lapses—essential for improvement. Punitive actions erode morale; ignoring or canceling delays perpetuates errors. Observation informs sustainable process redesign.
SubChapter: Quality Observation & Assessment

Q789. Answer: A

Explanation: Simplified electronic reporting increases submission rates and timeliness, improving trend analysis. Complex, lengthy, or restricted systems discourage participation. Accessibility and usability are key to promoting safety culture and transparent event learning.
SubChapter: Technology & Safety Systems

Q790. Answer: C

Explanation: Continuous audits, feedback, and reinforcement ensure adherence to PPE standards. One-time reminders lack impact, and ignoring errors fosters unsafe habits. Sustained compliance relies on visible monitoring and accountability integrated into safety culture.
SubChapter: Infection Control Compliance

Q791. Answer: A

Explanation: Reinforcing timeouts ensures adherence to safety checks and prevents procedural errors. Ignoring protocol normalization endangers patients, shortening timeouts removes safety redundancy, and anonymous reporting without direct correction delays change. Immediate reinforcement promotes accountability and consistent compliance.
SubChapter: Procedural Safety

Q792. Answer: A

Explanation: Simplified and standardized discharge instructions with visual aids reduce post-discharge medication confusion. Extending visits may not address comprehension; adding medications increases complexity; removing labels worsens errors. Clear written and verbal teaching supports safe self-management.
SubChapter: Patient Education & Safety

Q793. Answer: A

Explanation: Audits identify documentation gaps, error trends, and workflow inefficiencies, guiding staff education and process improvement. Punitive or concealed audits discourage participation, and limiting documentation undermines legal and clinical completeness. Continuous auditing builds quality assurance culture.
SubChapter: Quality Audit & Monitoring

Q794. Answer: D

Explanation: Adjusting assignments distributes workload equitably and prevents burnout, sustaining safety and morale. Criticism, delayed breaks, or ignoring stress heighten risk for errors and turnover. Supportive staffing reflects professional leadership and workforce retention strategy.
SubChapter: Workforce Management

Q795. Answer: A

Explanation: Direct demonstration with immediate feedback provides constructive learning, reinforces standards, and builds competence. Punishment discourages openness, ignoring allows error repetition, and delayed feedback misses teachable moments. Modeling fosters professional growth and safety compliance.
SubChapter: Competency Development

Q796. Answer: A

Explanation: Admitting and reporting an error promptly reflects ethical responsibility and supports transparency. Concealing or blaming others hinders learning and may compromise patient safety. Accountability builds team trust and promotes continuous improvement in practice quality.
SubChapter: Ethics & Accountability

Q797. Answer: A
Explanation: Standardized patient education ensures consistent, evidence-based guidance across all providers, enhancing comprehension and adherence. Rotation without uniformity increases confusion; delays or cancellations neglect patient safety and satisfaction. Consistency reduces misinformation and fosters reliability.
SubChapter: Patient Education Standardization
Q798. Answer: D
Explanation: Collecting baseline compliance data defines current performance and allows comparison after interventions. Random training or punishment without data undermines improvement, and ignoring data prevents measurable outcomes. Baseline assessment is essential for evidence-driven QI.
SubChapter: Quality Improvement Planning
Q799. Answer: A
Explanation: Presenting guideline-based evidence ensures clinical decisions remain objective and safe. Silence or bias erodes collaboration, and withdrawal disrupts communication. Evidence-driven advocacy models professionalism and upholds patient safety standards.
SubChapter: Interprofessional Collaboration
Q800. Answer: A
Explanation: Zero verification mismatches confirm adherence to safety protocols, reducing risk of adverse medication events. Charting speed, staffing patterns, and case volume are secondary operational metrics not reflective of process accuracy or safety quality.
SubChapter: Medication Verification & Safety

Questions (801-850)

Q801. A 48-year-old nurse feels pressured to administer chemo without a double-check due to staffing shortage. The correct professional action is to:
A. Refuse safely
B. Proceed anyway
C. Ignore policy
D. Request later

Q802. After a sentinel event, the unit schedules a debrief. What is the main purpose?
A. Protect image
B. Assign blame
C. Delay change
D. Identify causes

Q803. A quality report shows decreased compliance with PPE use. Which action should follow?
A. Conduct retraining
B. Lower standards
C. Skip audits
D. Ignore data

Q804. A new protocol reduces central line infections but increases workload. What should leadership prioritize?
A. Balance workload
B. Reverse policy
C. Ignore burden
D. Skip review

Q805. A nurse researcher analyzes transplant outcomes over three years. What type of study is this?
A. Retrospective
B. Prospective
C. Experimental
D. Anecdotal

Q806. A 32-year-old patient questions privacy during team discussions. What ensures ethical compliance?
A. Ignore request
B. Share broadly
C. Post details
D. Limit access

Q807. The unit's falls increased despite education efforts. What next step is most appropriate?
A. Reassess root
B. Repeat posters
C. Stop tracking
D. Shift blame

Q808. A nurse mentor encourages peers to present at conferences. This demonstrates:
A. Professional growth
B. Mandatory duty
C. Financial goal
D. Personal bias

Q809. A nurse updates patient teaching materials with current research. What quality Chapter does this represent?
A. Evidence translation

B. Risk avoidance
C. Cost reduction
D. Task delegation

Q810. A nurse preceptor observes inconsistent compliance with double-check policies among new hires. The best leadership step is to:
A. Ignore errors
B. Reinforce mentoring
C. Issue warning
D. Remove staff

Q811. A 59-year-old patient expresses concern about data privacy after consenting to research follow-up. The nurse's best response is to:
A. Explain protections
B. Minimize risk
C. Avoid details
D. Ignore query

Q812. During chart review, the nurse finds inconsistent documentation of fall risk scores. Which immediate action supports quality improvement?
A. Retrain staff
B. Erase notes
C. Delay audit
D. Ignore issue

Q813. A nurse observes colleagues using unapproved abbreviations. The appropriate action is to:
A. Educate staff
B. Report silently
C. Use same
D. Ignore trend

Q814. A staff nurse joins a committee reviewing patient safety events. What is the main benefit?
A. Less work
B. Higher pay
C. Shared learning
D. Social time

Q815. A 48-year-old nurse reports emotional exhaustion from frequent critical cases. The manager's best initial step is to:
A. Offer counseling
B. Add shifts
C. Dismiss stress
D. Reprimand nurse

Q816. A transplant nurse participates in an external benchmarking study. What primary goal does this activity serve?
A. Compare outcomes
B. Gain credit
C. Increase pay
D. Reduce staff

Q817. A patient experiences a medication delay because the barcoding system was offline. What should the team do?
A. Document and report
B. Administer blindly
C. Skip dose entirely

D. Hide incident

Q818. A nurse notes that some staff skip PPE due to time pressure. What improvement action is best?

A. Delay reminder
B. Add paperwork
C. Conduct audit
D. Remove policy

Q819. A 35-year-old patient expresses frustration about repetitive education from multiple nurses. The best quality improvement strategy is to:

A. Standardize teaching
B. Rotate randomly
C. Shorten sessions
D. Reduce documentation

Q820. A nurse reviews hospital incident data revealing increased falls at night. The first step toward resolution should be:

A. Analyze staffing
B. Replace floors
C. Punish staff
D. Delay response

Q821. A new BMT nurse hesitates to question a physician's unsafe order. What professional standard applies here?

A. Duty to advocate
B. Blind obedience
C. Silent compliance
D. Role avoidance

Q822. A nurse leader introduces a mentorship program for novice transplant nurses. The expected benefit is:

A. Less feedback
B. Lower morale
C. Higher retention
D. Reduced skill

Q823. A 56-year-old patient receives complex discharge instructions. To confirm comprehension, the nurse should:

A. Use teach-back
B. Hand pamphlet
C. Ask "okay?"
D. Skip review

Q824. A transplant unit plans to implement a new electronic medication record. What ensures smooth transition?

A. Staff training
B. Sudden rollout
C. Minimal input
D. No feedback

Q825. A nurse develops a checklist for blood transfusion verification. The main expected outcome is:

A. Error reduction
B. Faster discharge
C. Higher census
D. Less charting

Q826. A nurse manager introduces peer review to enhance clinical practice. What defines a successful program?
A. Punitive focus
B. Public criticism
C. Constructive feedback
D. Random scoring
Q827. A 50-year-old nurse reports confusion about ethical guidelines for informed consent. The educator should emphasize:
A. Patient autonomy
B. Staff hierarchy
C. Institutional loyalty
D. Time efficiency
Q828. During a leadership meeting, data reveal rising medication discrepancies. The first collective step should be to:
A. Conduct root cause
B. Assign blame
C. Hide results
D. Delay action
Q829. A nurse manager notices poor attendance in safety training sessions. Which intervention best improves participation?
A. Flexible scheduling
B. Mandatory penalties
C. No reminders
D. Cancel sessions
Q830. A nurse reviews monthly central line infection data showing consistent improvement. What is the next appropriate step?
A. Halt education
B. End audits
C. Relax standards
D. Sustain gains
Q831. A nurse educator prepares a workshop on error prevention. The most effective teaching strategy is:
A. Use case studies
B. Read policies
C. Skip examples
D. Avoid questions
Q832. During a high workload shift, a nurse decides to bypass double-checks for chemotherapy. The appropriate managerial response is to:
A. Address promptly
B. Ignore choice
C. Delay review
D. Punish harshly
Q833. A 44-year-old patient questions why safety checklists are repeated multiple times daily. The nurse should respond by:
A. Explaining purpose
B. Reducing checks
C. Avoiding reply
D. Skipping steps

Q834. A nurse manager notes increased overtime among staff. The best first action to ensure safety is to:
A. Add shifts
B. Ignore data
C. Assess workload
D. Cut pay
Q835. A post-transplant patient refuses a required isolation protocol. What is the nurse's next appropriate step?
A. Provide rationale
B. Enforce quietly
C. Ignore refusal
D. Report instantly
Q836. A nurse audits charting accuracy after new EMR implementation. Which finding indicates success?
A. Fewer omissions
B. Extra pages
C. More clicks
D. Less access
Q837. A new staff nurse hesitates to participate in morbidity review meetings. The preceptor should emphasize that such meetings:
A. Promote learning
B. Punish errors
C. Shame staff
D. Assign guilt
Q838. A transplant unit tracks adherence to central line protocols monthly. This represents which quality activity?
A. Staff ranking
B. Random survey
C. Process monitoring
D. Event gossip
Q839. A nurse leader seeks to reduce variance in discharge summary completion times. The most effective tool is:
A. Flow diagram
B. Staff memo
C. Random guess
D. Quick fix
Q840. During quality rounds, a nurse notes expired medications in a crash cart. The correct immediate action is to:
A. Remove items
B. Record later
C. Ignore issue
D. Blame staff
Q841. A patient's caregiver reports receiving conflicting dietary information. The most effective leadership response is to:
A. Standardize content
B. Shift blame
C. Ignore concern
D. Add random tips

Q842. A nurse participates in creating a falls-prevention checklist. This involvement primarily promotes:
A. Silence
B. Resistance
C. Indifference
D. Ownership
Q843. After an audit, the nurse identifies poor documentation of blood transfusion consent. The next step should be to:
A. Provide education
B. Hide findings
C. Delay action
D. Blame staff
Q844. A nurse receives feedback about incomplete shift handoff reports. The most professional response is to:
A. Improve practice
B. Deny issue
C. Blame others
D. Avoid change
Q845. A nurse-led project decreases CLABSI rates by 40%. To maintain success, the team should:
A. Continue monitoring
B. Stop audits
C. Relax policy
D. Reduce staff
Q846. A 39-year-old nurse advocates for standardized chemotherapy administration policies. This demonstrates:
A. Apathy
B. Obedience
C. Resistance
D. Leadership
Q847. After a patient fall, the nurse completes an incident report. The primary purpose of this action is to:
A. Improve safety
B. Punish staff
C. Assign blame
D. Hide data
Q848. A nurse manager introduces simulation drills for emergency response training. The expected benefit is:
A. Improved readiness
B. Lower morale
C. Increased confusion
D. Delayed action
Q849. A 47-year-old BMT nurse wants to publish a case report on GVHD management. The first step is to:
A. Obtain consent
B. Write freely
C. Skip approval
D. Hide details

Q850. A nurse observes that many peers avoid reporting near-misses. The most effective strategy to change behavior is to:

A. Ignore gaps
B. Threaten punishment
C. Promote openness
D. Delay feedback

Answer key and Explanation (801-850)
Q801. Answer: A
Explanation: Refusing unsafe orders preserves patient safety and professional integrity, complying with institutional and legal standards. Proceeding without verification endangers patients, violates policy, and exposes liability. Safe refusal exemplifies ethical nursing judgment.
SubChapter: Ethical Decision-Making
Q802. Answer: D
Explanation: Post-event debriefs identify root causes, strengthen learning, and guide preventive strategies. Blame or image protection hinders open dialogue, and delays reduce relevance. Transparent reflection transforms adverse events into improvement opportunities.
SubChapter: Event Debriefing & Learning
Q803. Answer: A
Explanation: Retraining reinforces correct techniques and accountability while addressing knowledge gaps. Lowering standards or halting audits diminishes safety, and ignoring findings perpetuates risk. Active education restores compliance and strengthens infection prevention culture.
SubChapter: Compliance & Infection Safety
Q804. Answer: A
Explanation: Balancing workload maintains safety gains while protecting staff well-being. Reversal discards progress, ignoring strain risks burnout, and skipping review misses optimization opportunities. Sustainable quality improvement requires clinical and workforce balance.
SubChapter: Quality Sustainability
Q805. Answer: A
Explanation: Retrospective studies review existing data to identify trends and associations. Prospective studies collect future data; experimental trials involve interventions; anecdotal reports lack systematic methodology. Retrospective analysis supports evidence-based quality enhancement.
SubChapter: Research & Evidence Evaluation
Q806. Answer: D
Explanation: Limiting data access to authorized personnel protects patient confidentiality and aligns with HIPAA and ethical codes. Broad sharing, public posting, or disregard for privacy violates legal and professional obligations. Confidentiality maintains trust and dignity.
SubChapter: Patient Rights & Confidentiality
Q807. Answer: A
Explanation: Reassessing root causes identifies deeper contributors—staffing, environment, or patient acuity—that education alone missed. Repetition without analysis wastes effort; ignoring or blaming prevents resolution. Continuous assessment fosters adaptive improvement.
SubChapter: QI Reassessment
Q808. Answer: A
Explanation: Promoting scholarly engagement strengthens professional development, knowledge sharing, and leadership visibility. It is voluntary, not mandatory, and unrelated to personal gain. Encouragement fosters continual learning and evidence dissemination.
SubChapter: Professional Development
Q809. Answer: A
Explanation: Integrating new evidence into patient materials reflects translation of research into practice, enhancing relevance and effectiveness. Risk management and cost are indirect benefits, and delegation is unrelated. Evidence translation maintains clinical quality alignment.
SubChapter: Evidence-Based Improvement
Q810. Answer: B

Explanation: Mentoring and coaching correct noncompliance constructively, ensuring understanding and sustainability. Punishment without education discourages openness, and removal or ignorance fails to address learning needs. Reinforcement builds safe and consistent practice habits.
SubChapter: Leadership & Mentorship

Q811. Answer: A

Explanation: Explaining confidentiality procedures (coding, secure databases, restricted access) reassures patients and demonstrates ethical transparency. Minimization or avoidance undermines trust, and ignoring concerns violates informed consent standards and ethical nursing practice.
SubChapter: Research Ethics & Patient Rights

Q812. Answer: A

Explanation: Retraining reinforces standardized scoring, ensuring accuracy and reliability of fall prevention data. Erasing records breaches integrity; delays allow continued error; ignoring perpetuates unsafe trends. Education aligns team documentation for effective risk monitoring.
SubChapter: Documentation Accuracy & QI

Q813. Answer: A

Explanation: Providing immediate education promotes safe communication and prevents medication or treatment errors. Silent reporting without guidance delays correction, copying errors spreads risk, and ignorance violates documentation policy. Continuous reminders sustain compliance.
SubChapter: Communication Standards & Safety

Q814. Answer: C

Explanation: Committee participation promotes multidisciplinary learning, builds analytical skills, and embeds safety awareness in daily practice. Monetary or workload motives are secondary, and treating committees as social spaces undermines professional purpose.
SubChapter: Team Engagement in Safety

Q815. Answer: A

Explanation: Offering access to counseling or peer support addresses compassion fatigue and prevents burnout. Adding workload or dismissing emotions risks errors and attrition, while reprimand discourages transparency. Support sustains workforce mental health and safety culture.
SubChapter: Workforce Wellness & Retention

Q816. Answer: A

Explanation: Benchmarking compares performance against peer institutions, identifying improvement opportunities and best practices. Personal or financial incentives are secondary. Comparative analysis drives data-informed decisions and elevates care quality standards.
SubChapter: Quality Benchmarking

Q817. Answer: A

Explanation: Documenting and reporting system downtime ensures patient safety tracking and IT correction. Administering without verification increases risk, skipping doses disrupts therapy, and concealment prevents systemic improvement. Reporting preserves transparency and accountability.
SubChapter: Technology & Safety

Q818. Answer: C

Explanation: Auditing compliance identifies behavior patterns, barriers, and knowledge gaps. Paperwork or delay reinforces noncompliance; removing PPE policy contradicts infection prevention. Audit-driven feedback and education restore adherence to safety standards.
SubChapter: Compliance Monitoring

Q819. Answer: A

Explanation: Standardizing education ensures consistency and prevents mixed messages, improving patient satisfaction and retention. Random rotation and shortened sessions risk incomplete understanding; reducing documentation removes verification of teaching effectiveness.

SubChapter: Patient Education Quality

Q820. Answer: A

Explanation: Staffing analysis examines adequacy, skill mix, and supervision during high-risk hours. Facility changes or punishment lack evidence linkage, and delay prolongs risk. Rooted staffing evaluation addresses underlying system imbalance effectively.

SubChapter: Data-Driven Safety Assessment

Q821. Answer: A

Explanation: Nurses are ethically bound to advocate for patient safety by questioning or clarifying unsafe orders. Obedience without verification or silence endangers care, and avoidance neglects professional accountability. Advocacy ensures ethical practice and patient trust.

SubChapter: Professional Ethics & Advocacy

Q822. Answer: C

Explanation: Mentorship promotes skill growth, job satisfaction, and retention by fostering support and continuous learning. Poor morale and limited feedback occur without mentorship. Programs strengthen confidence and reduce early turnover in high-acuity units.

SubChapter: Mentorship & Retention

Q823. Answer: A

Explanation: Teach-back validates patient understanding by requiring demonstration or verbal explanation, ensuring safety and reducing readmission risk. Pamphlets alone are passive, brief confirmation questions insufficient, and omission neglects education standards.

SubChapter: Patient Education & Safety

Q824. Answer: A

Explanation: Comprehensive training prepares users, reduces errors, and builds confidence. Abrupt implementation without feedback causes resistance and documentation issues. Continuous training supports workflow adaptation and successful adoption.

SubChapter: Technology Implementation & Quality

Q825. Answer: A

Explanation: Checklists standardize high-risk procedures, preventing mismatches and human errors. Operational outcomes like discharge speed or census do not measure safety success. Structured verification ensures patient identity and transfusion accuracy.

SubChapter: Safety Tools & Standardization

Q826. Answer: C

Explanation: Constructive peer feedback identifies growth areas while maintaining respect and confidentiality. Public or punitive reviews discourage participation, and random scoring lacks validity. Positive peer review strengthens accountability and performance consistency.

SubChapter: Peer Review & Professional Growth

Q827. Answer: A

Explanation: Informed consent prioritizes patient autonomy, ensuring understanding and voluntary decision-making. Institutional or time pressures cannot override ethical duty to patient-centered communication. Respect for autonomy safeguards dignity and legal integrity.

SubChapter: Ethics & Patient Autonomy

Q828. Answer: A

Explanation: Root cause analysis uncovers process failures contributing to medication discrepancies, guiding corrective interventions. Blame and concealment destroy trust and transparency; delaying action allows continued risk. Systematic evaluation yields lasting improvement.

SubChapter: Medication Safety & RCA

Q829. Answer: A

Explanation: Flexible session scheduling accommodates staff shifts, improving attendance and engagement. Penalties discourage learning, lack of reminders lowers participation, and cancellation removes vital education. Adaptability encourages sustained safety culture compliance.
SubChapter: Education & Engagement Strategies

Q830. Answer: D

Explanation: Sustaining improvement requires ongoing monitoring, recognition, and reinforcement of best practices. Ending audits or relaxing standards risks regression, while ceasing education erodes compliance. Sustainability maintains achieved outcomes long term.
SubChapter: Quality Maintenance & Sustainability

Q831. Answer: A

Explanation: Case studies connect concepts to real practice, allowing reflection and learning from near-misses or adverse events. Reading policies alone limits engagement, while skipping discussion reduces understanding. Interactive methods improve knowledge retention and safety behavior.
SubChapter: Education & Learning Strategy

Q832. Answer: A

Explanation: Immediate, supportive feedback emphasizes safety standards and explores systemic causes of bypassing checks. Ignoring or delaying responses enables recurrence; punitive reactions create fear. Timely intervention fosters accountability and process redesign for safety compliance.
SubChapter: Leadership & Safety Enforcement

Q833. Answer: A

Explanation: Explaining that repetition ensures consistency and prevents critical errors enhances patient trust. Reducing or skipping steps compromises safety, and avoidance diminishes confidence. Transparency validates the role of redundancy in high-risk transplant care.
SubChapter: Patient Communication & Safety

Q834. Answer: C

Explanation: Workload assessment identifies resource or process inefficiencies causing excessive overtime, preventing fatigue-related errors. Ignoring or exacerbating workload undermines quality. Addressing root workload causes preserves well-being and patient safety.
SubChapter: Workforce Management

Q835. Answer: A

Explanation: Explaining the purpose and consequences of isolation fosters understanding and voluntary cooperation. Silent enforcement or ignoring resistance violates autonomy and safety; premature reporting without discussion prevents resolution. Education builds compliance through respect and clarity.
SubChapter: Patient Rights & Safety

Q836. Answer: A

Explanation: Reduced omissions and complete data entry reflect improved EMR utilization and documentation accuracy. Interface complexity or increased clicks are usability factors but not indicators of quality. Comprehensive charting supports patient safety and compliance.
SubChapter: Technology Integration & Quality

Q837. Answer: A

Explanation: Morbidity reviews aim to analyze cases objectively for learning and prevention, not punishment. Fear-based perceptions hinder participation. Framing meetings as collaborative opportunities builds transparency and continuous improvement culture.
SubChapter: Safety & Review Culture

Q838. Answer: C

Explanation: Monitoring protocol adherence evaluates real-time compliance with established safety procedures. Surveys or gossip lack structure, and ranking introduces bias. Regular monitoring sustains high performance and early detection of deviations.
SubChapter: Quality Measurement
Q839. Answer: A
Explanation: Flow diagrams map discharge processes to locate bottlenecks and streamline documentation. Memos or guesswork lack data basis, while quick fixes fail to address systemic issues. Visualization drives process redesign.
SubChapter: Process Analysis
Q840. Answer: A
Explanation: Immediate removal of expired medications prevents potential harm, followed by documentation and restocking. Ignoring or blaming delays correction and weakens accountability. Quick remediation aligns with safety standards.
SubChapter: Medication Management & Safety
Q841. Answer: A
Explanation: Standardizing dietary education ensures accuracy, consistency, and alignment with medical recommendations. Blame and neglect foster confusion; arbitrary tips worsen inconsistency. Structured education enhances patient trust and adherence.
SubChapter: Education Consistency
Q842. Answer: D
Explanation: Engaging staff in quality design fosters ownership, accountability, and higher compliance rates. Excluding nurses causes detachment and weakens intervention success. Participation builds a shared commitment to safety goals.
SubChapter: Staff Engagement in QI
Q843. Answer: A
Explanation: Targeted education corrects knowledge gaps and reinforces consent documentation standards. Concealment or blame diminishes improvement potential, and delay increases risk. Educational remediation promotes compliance and ethical care.
SubChapter: Documentation & Ethics
Q844. Answer: A
Explanation: Accepting feedback constructively and addressing gaps demonstrates accountability and commitment to safe communication. Denial or blame prevents improvement; avoidance sustains risk. Professional reflection supports growth and teamwork.
SubChapter: Communication & Accountability
Q845. Answer: A
Explanation: Ongoing monitoring verifies sustained compliance and reinforces best practices. Stopping oversight or relaxing rules risks reversal of progress. Consistent feedback ensures long-term infection control success.
SubChapter: Quality Maintenance
Q846. Answer: D
Explanation: Advocating for standardization shows initiative and dedication to safety and evidence-based care. Passive or resistant attitudes hinder system improvement. Leadership fosters collaboration and continuous advancement of practice standards.
SubChapter: Professional Leadership
Q847. Answer: A
Explanation: Incident reporting enables system analysis, identification of contributing factors, and targeted prevention strategies. Punishment or concealment prevents learning, while transparency ensures proactive safety measures.

SubChapter: Incident Reporting & Learning

Q848. Answer: A

Explanation: Simulation builds confidence and teamwork, improving staff readiness during real emergencies. It enhances coordination and identifies system gaps. Negative outcomes occur only without structure; proper drills strengthen performance and safety.

SubChapter: Emergency Preparedness

Q849. Answer: A

Explanation: Patient consent is mandatory before publishing identifiable information, ensuring ethical and legal compliance. Writing without approval or concealment violates confidentiality. Transparency supports professional integrity and trust.

SubChapter: Research & Publication Ethics

Q850. Answer: C

Explanation: Promoting an open, nonpunitive culture encourages staff to report near-misses, fostering proactive risk management. Punitive approaches and neglect reinforce underreporting. Transparent leadership drives continuous safety improvement.

SubChapter: Safety Culture & Transparency

Made in United States
Orlando, FL
04 November 2026

90201061R00122